STOP
HIDING
BEHIND YOUR
WEIGHT

The Spiritually Intelligent
Woman's Guide to Releasing
Physical and Emotional
Weight

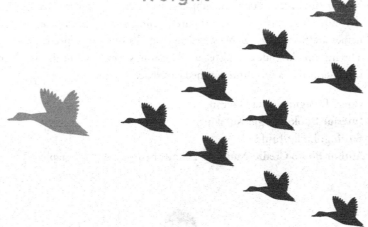

PO-HONG YU, LAc

STOP HIDING BEHIND YOUR WEIGHT

The Spiritually Intelligent Woman's Guide to Releasing Physical and Emotional Weight

Difference Press, Washington, D.C., USA
© Po-Hong Yu, LAc, 2021

ISBN: 978-1-68309-298-8

Cover Design: Nakita Duncan
Interior Book Design: Kozakura
Editing: Emily Tuttle
Author Photo Credit: Nancy La Lanne of La Lanne Photography

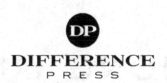

DIFFERENCE PRESS

To the three loves I grieved,
in the last three months,
that catapulted this book into creation.
In great pain lives even greater possibilities.

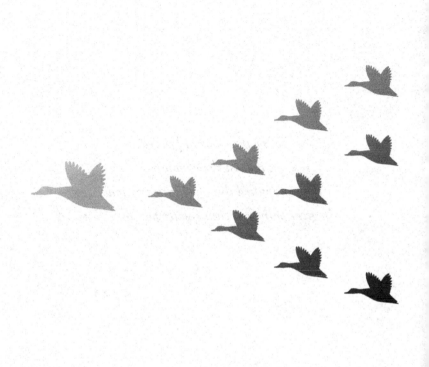

TABLE OF CONTENTS

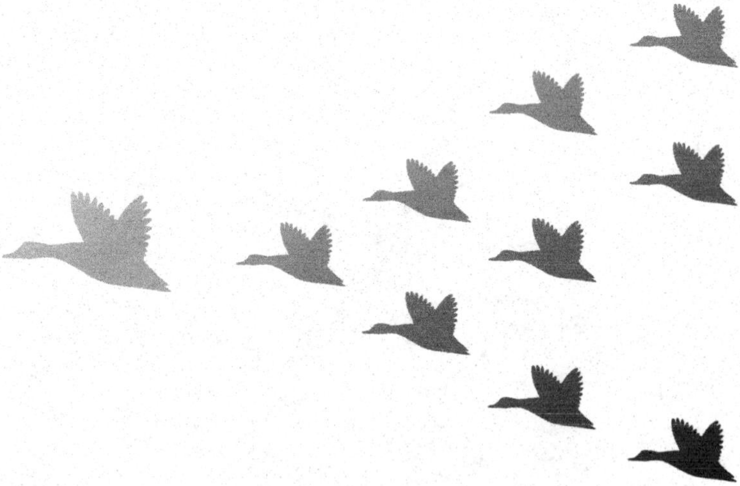

FOREWORD

Despite being 5'2" and 130 pounds, Po is larger than life. She's funny, irreverent, deeply curious, and relentless in her pursuit of truth, health, and resilience. She eats mangos with gusto, has a wild, contagious laugh, and loves nothing more than feeling fully alive no matter what she's experiencing – a heart-wrenching tsunami in the wake of a loss or an unexpected joy. She's one of those people you can trust deeply, because what's inside her is visible in her eyes and face, tone of voice, and gestures. She weeps when she's sad, shares her anger directly, loves fiercely, and isn't above asking for help when she's in pain.

Po and I met several years ago when we sat next to each other by chance in the audience of a women's empowerment program in New York City. Within a few moments of introducing ourselves, we were talking about our darkest fears and deepest desires. "I want to come out of hiding, to serve the world on a bigger scale," I remember her telling me. "But I'm used to being invisible in plain sight. That's part of my experience, particularly as an Asian-American woman." Po wastes no time. She jumps right into the heart of things, and has the courage to risk the potential blowback of other people's reactions when there's a healing opportunity at hand.

To me, this is part of what makes her a modern-day visionary healer. In this book, you'll get a taste of her gifts. She won't take you anywhere she hasn't been first, and she won't watch from the sidelines, giving detached guidance. She's more of a knee-deep, roll-up-your-sleeves, no-holds-barred type of teacher who gets right up in there with you, whether in person, online, or here, in this book. She's humble and real, because she wants the same thing for all women who hide to protect themselves – more healing. More vitality. More you.

Po's weight loss program is unusual because it's not actually about losing anything. It's about gaining yourself – your true self. It's a program that has much more to do with remembering who you are than with becoming someone you think you want to be. Po brings her own unique, holistic approach to the body and to healing physical and emotional symptoms of distress. As an acupuncturist who has worked for years helping others resolve intractable physical and emotional pain issues, and as the daughter of a Taoist spiritual teacher, her understanding of the mind-body-spirit connection is practical and intuitive.

In this book, she weaves her own personal wisdom and experience as a woman and healer with important concepts drawn from Taoism, eastern philosophy, and a variety of different psychological frameworks, with a dash of wry Brooklynite humor thrown in for good measure. She keeps her teachings and guidance relevant, grounded in our modern world. Her passion for helping women reconnect with balance and flow is palpable on every page.

In *Stop Hiding behind Your Weight*, you'll learn how being smart and successful in many areas of your life can get in the way of your own healing. You'll also be guided to harness your gifts, creativity, and generosity in new and powerful ways, using them to shed physical and emotional weight that has served as "body armor" protecting you from pain while simultaneously keeping you constricted and blocked. You'll be introduced to valuable tools and practices that will help you expand into greater freedom, and develop a more loving relationship with yourself.

As you read this book, I have no doubt you'll get a sense of Po's commitment to helping you heal, and be inspired by it. She'll go the distance with you, and support you in finding your own answers, all while respecting that your journey is yours to choose.

Alicia Muñoz, LPC

Author of *No More Fighting* and *A Year of Us*

Po-Hong has written a game-changing book for women who are struggling with weight loss. With the courage of a warrior, she cuts through all the bullsh*t and teaches the reader to process the hurt, pain, and longing that must be addressed for a woman to have a healthy relationship with her body. Her work as an acupuncturist allows her to understand the root cause of imbalances and solve them. This book is a victory march for body love!

Regena Thomashauer (a.k.a. "Mama Gena")

is a teacher and best-selling author of *Pussy: A Reclamation,* and the founder and CEO of the School of Womanly Arts.

CHAPTER 1

THE FINAL FRONTIER

"I had on a fifty-pound emotional jacket... The cost of that jacket was my personal joy and a good night's sleep. I decided to begin shedding the jacket and take back all my power."
— Lisa Nichols

Maybe you know her. She's the woman in the self-help aisle of the bookstore, always seeking. She's sitting in the front and back rows of personal development courses, taking notes, having epiphanies, trying to get better, trying to feel better. She's done so much work, made so much progress, realized so many things and yet she's still stuck in a body she resents, ignores, and dislikes. Her body feels heavy. It's as if she's carrying within it much more than just physical weight. She's also carrying the weight of unfelt losses, of unexpressed hurts, of a lifetime of emotional pain. Much of the time, she feels like she'd rather not be seen. Why? What good could come from being seen? Attention feels unsafe. Sometimes, it's as if she's afraid of meeting herself, her real self underneath all of the hiding.

This woman was me. Maybe she's also you? I did so much emotional and spiritual work but still hid behind my body armor. I have to admit it was a brilliant self-protection tactic, one I see all the time in so many women; women who are successful and happy for the most part, but who are also using the avoidance or denial of their unreleased weight as a protective mechanism. This holds them back from connecting to who they really are underneath it all. They overcompensate for their lack of consciousness around their body with their abilities and gifts in supporting, nurturing, or taking care of others. In a sense, the shedding of this weight and the reasons why they have this body armor to begin with is their final frontier.

Even if you have done tons of personal development work and read all of the self-help books, it is still possible to be stuck in an area that holds the most fear. So, it's important not to judge or admonish yourself. I'm guessing you have been focusing on your emotional healing but avoiding your body. Is that true? That's certainly what I did. I went deeply into healing the emotional elements of my past trauma and I got stuck there. I over processed, or at least I thought I was processing, but later realized I was indulging in overthinking, worrying, and obsessing. I was comfortable in this space because I was addicted to suffering (which is very different than truly feeling your emotions). I was in tune with high levels of perception and had a profound knowledge of various philosophies, but they had no grounding in my body. I couldn't *live* them. "Emotional work" and spirituality were my comfort zones, and I used these to disconnect from both my mind and body.

The body aspect was more obvious: I lacked consciousness in eating, avoided exercise, wore clothes that felt safe, checked in and out during sex, and in general, disconnected physically in almost every area of my life.

But with the mind, it was a bit trickier. I found myself being too smart for my own good. Do you relate to this? I was emotionally intelligent, empathic, and intuitive, *but* I allowed my ego to completely run the show. I obsessed about everything. I worried about what people thought of me all the time. I future-tripped about things I couldn't control. I ruminated on everything that had happened to me in the past. Basically, I was unable to see that I built a lifelong practice of choosing suffering and drama instead of seeing things as they actually were. And as a result, lying dormant, was a ton of unprocessed emotions I had never fully felt, nor allowed myself to heal from. I thought I was processing them but, little did I know, what I was actually doing was bypassing them.

I believe that this a common denominator for all humans, but I have noticed an interesting phenomenon; and it is this: women, and often women who are sensitive, intelligent, and aware often use their intelligence, sensitivity and awareness to *avoid* their own healing. Crazy, isn't it? There are many women out there who are spiritual seekers and high achievers, who have achieved success in many areas of their lives, but have yet to release the weight they have been carrying for years. It doesn't mean you have done anything wrong or that you didn't get something right. It just means that you have been focusing on specific areas that are comfortable for you while ignoring the others. For many of us, the weight we haven't released is our blind spot. We end up subconsciously hypnotizing ourselves against our truest desires.

SURVIVAL MODE

When we go through traumatic experiences, especially at an early age, we create a sense of safety that may not necessarily be healthy but is definitely effective. We learn to numb and disconnect from our bodies, or even disassociate from even having a body, as I did. Our nervous system has one priority – to keep us safe. If creating layers of fat was the way you did that, then congratulations, you are a genius! Because the other option was unimaginably painful, and your younger self probably wouldn't have been able to survive emotionally. Perhaps she wouldn't have gotten through school, or she would've had a complete mental breakdown, or she would've hurt herself in much greater emotional or physical ways.

This may sound dramatic, but what you did instinctually was a survival mechanism. You probably didn't have any tools to process your emotions. Most adults haven't been taught healthy ways to process trauma or emotions, so you can imagine what it's like for a kid.

It makes perfect sense to gain weight because our bodies are our inherent protection. If someone physically attacks you, all you have is your body as a defense. The reptilian part of our brain reacts instinctively when danger appears. This is often referred to as our freeze-flight-fight mode. But our emotional bodies have learned how to protect us too. The number of women that have been traumatized by physical, sexual, emotional, and cultural abuse is astronomical and, I believe, is in direct correlation to why some women carry extra weight as a protective mechanism.

Just look at the statistics: One in five women have been raped at some point in her life and those are just numbers that have been reported! I never reported my rapes, and many, many other women have not reported theirs either. In my personal experience, which you will read about in the next chapter, I immediately gained weight after my first rape. I didn't have any awareness about what was happening at the time, but it's clear when looking back at my childhood photos, and at my psyche, that through gaining weight, I was trying to protect myself.

Sexual, physical, and emotional abuse are obvious forms of trauma. But there are other forms that aren't as obvious, but have wounds that cut just as deep. Cultural expectations and judgments can cause the same traumatic impact on us, but they are more subtle and travel in the undertones of culture.

For example, white privilege and the patriarchy have created generations of internalized self-judgements and shame, and affect how most women relate to their bodies. Women have been conditioned to think that having a thin lighter-skinned body is the ideal, and if you don't, you are not as sexy, sensual, or beautiful as those who do. This is communicated in many ways, such as in media and films. When, on top of that, you add living in a body that has been historically seen and treated as something less than human or at the bottom of the barrel, it becomes an even more traumatic experience. Women of color, queer and trans people, and disabled people have all learned from a young age that they are not anywhere close to society's gold standard, and in return, they tend to internalize these messages as self-hatred. This is precisely what happened to me, being a queer, first generation Chinese American; and then, because I hated myself, I tried to mold myself in an attempt to become anyone but myself.

The unconscious mind is powerful and will do anything to protect us, even if it hurts us in other ways. Protection is the number one priority of our unconscious minds, and hiding behind our weight is actually a brilliant method of protection. It is common knowledge that both animals and armies use camouflage as a defense tactic. Humans can do exactly the same thing with extra weight.

HIDING

When most people think about hiding, they are talking about hiding from the outside world due to feeling unsafe. Being afraid of the male gaze while walking down the street, being visible, promoting your business on social media, or afraid to date and allow a potential lover or partner into your most vulnerable and intimate spaces. This is common and was definitely the case for me.

But the truth is that anything that we feel about the outside world is a projection of our internal world.

My weight kept me from getting to know the real me. I could always feel a part of me deep inside that wanted to come out, but I couldn't access it, and frankly, it felt safer not letting her out. I was afraid to meet the woman behind my fear fat suit, a woman who was radiant, powerful, confident, free, and connectable. I surmised that if I lost the physical and emotional weight, it meant I would be "forced" to create the life I desired, and I would have to show up in new and uncomfortable ways that I didn't trust that I couldn't handle or sustain, or worse, that once achieved, I could lose at a moment's notice.

I believe that our biggest fear is actually having what we want in life, because actually *having* what we want is all unknown territory. It's so much safer to live in a place of comfort, to avoid risking rejection, to avoid loss, to hide from real and lasting transformation and change.

MARTYRDOM & BOUNDARIES

Another possible outcome of trauma is being confused about boundaries. We may not understand how healthy boundaries are developed or how to work with them in relating to others. When our own boundaries have been violated, we may pick up the belief that our bodies don't really belong to us and are not valuable or worthy. That's when some women create a weight buffer. Since we were unable to connect with our power and use our voice to say 'no' during vulnerable and fearful experiences, we find another way to say 'no' - through our bodies. We come to the conclusion that if we can make ourselves less desirable, perhaps we won't be sexually violated again. Or if we gain weight, maybe we will just disappear into the background and our parents, teachers, or other important adults in our lives won't abuse us because they won't even see us. We'll be invisible.

In our inability to connect with our authentic and true voice, when requests or demands are made of us, we learn to prioritize other people's needs and to focus on taking care of them rather than taking care of ourselves. Often, because we lack self-esteem and self-worth, we try to find value in our lives through caretaking, people-pleasing, or fixing. You may have convinced yourself that you're a good person for all of the good deeds you've done but the truth is that you are using your habit of focusing on other people to escape yourself. It is an absolutely genius and common tactic; it blows up your ego to give you a false sense of worth, but in reality, it's just a Band-Aid, and a flimsy one at that.

After my rapes, I would give all of me away, whether it was money, my time, attention, energy, sex, or through caretaking. I already felt like a piece of disposable trash since my body was treated that way, so I behaved accordingly. I acted as if my life were not my own. Looking at me from the outside, you never would have thought I was doing this because I worked hard to perfect the role of a fiery and outspoken woman. But behind this facade, I was terrified of real connection. This deep sense of lacking and disconnection from myself was a mask, and it perpetuated a very codependent way of living.

Are you always trying to save, rescue, or fix someone or something? It may seem like you are trying to do good and you may think you mean well but really, you are chasing a distorted form of control because you feel so out of control on the inside. You may want to save other people because you're the one who really wants to be saved. You may get your sense of worth from helping others because you're unable to feel your innate worthiness. You may feel that you are ultimately responsible for other people's suffering and wellbeing. If so, your behavior is that of a martyr. This is tricky because you are convinced that you are doing good out of the kindness of your heart, but underneath it all, you are searching for love and a sense of value. You may not be giving from a place of self-love and fullness. Instead, you are giving to get.

SELF-SABOTAGE

Do you feel comfortable in the skin you're in?

Do you like what you see in the mirror?

Do you even look at yourself in the mirror?

Do you base your beauty off of what society says is beautiful, or do you have your own personal definition of beauty?

So many women I've talked to have admitted that they have attempted to release the weight so many times that they have lost their trust in themselves. Their fear of failure keeps them stuck in a cycle of feeling 'not good enough' and also of feeling fundamentally powerless to release the extra weight they have been hiding behind. Do you relate? Have you been in a cycle of weight-releasing "failures?" Do you feel like you are at least to some degree clueless when it comes to knowing what your body needs because you have lived for so many years being so disconnected from it?

When you hide behind your weight, even if your life is great in every other way, you most likely don't feel truly satisfied or fulfilled within yourself. You probably have that nagging feeling that there's a gaping hole of emptiness because your resistance to truly taking care of yourself and releasing the weight creates more suffering. There's a part of you that feels dead and numb inside, even if you are, by most measures, a fairly happy person. I wanted to be more than fairly happy. I wanted to feel alive! I wanted to feel turned-on and juicy. I wanted something far beyond mediocre. I wanted to live my best life.

I'm guessing you're reading this book because you're sick of avoiding certain parts of yourself. You're probably secretly telling yourself that you can't have everything you want because it's scarier to have the life you desire than not. That is called self-sabotage, and it's more common than you may realize. Self-sabotage happens when you subconsciously make a deal with yourself to stay in your comfort zone so that when you get to a certain level of success, your subconscious mind finds a way to bring you back down to familiar territory. If you look at your life and think about the times that you started to achieve success in a certain area, or received something that you really desired, you may have self-sabotaged shortly afterwards. The funny thing about self-sabotage is that it unconsciously happens in any and all ways that you can possibly imagine. Here are a few examples:

- You finally scored a meeting with the CEO, and then you get extremely ill and can't make it.
- You fall madly in love with someone, and as soon as they talk about marriage, you create a huge fight and then break up (this was my brilliant way of sabotaging relationships).
- You start to release the weight and feel good in your body and then start overeating again and gain all the weight back plus an extra few pounds.

If you want to learn more about unconscious sabotage patterns, check out the book, "The Big Leap" by Gay Hendricks. He calls the process "upper-limiting" and it is a real eye-opener.

THE POSSIBILITIES

If any or all of this chapter resonated with you, congratulations! You are a master saboteur! Now it's time for the next phase of your life where you consciously choose how you want to live because you are now able to see there is a different path.

This new way of living doesn't involve hiding anymore. The new way is about living an embodied life, *on purpose*, with confidence and connection to your highest self and to others. It is about feeling sensual and sexy in your body. It is about the ability to radiate a cultivated 'turn-on' out into the world through your work, your relationships, your very essence, while walking down the street or just looking at yourself in the mirror.

It's one thing to be aligned in one or two realms of your life, but it's another thing to be aligned in all areas. When all three realms (emotional, mental, physical) receive the loving attention they deserve, everything *clicks* and energetic flow ensues! There is no stopping you because you are now self-realizing. This happens effortlessly when you are able to completely feel the power of the divine come swooping in to show you why you are here and proceed to guide you toward each next right step on your path. A sense of clarity and purpose enters, and a fullness of love inside prevails. You gain an awareness that you are living your best life and ready to take the quantum leaps into what you've always known, somewhere deep inside, that your biggest dreams are possible. Even if you've "forgotten," that vision is still living in a place within you. The dreamer in you lives, and when you choose to express the highest level of your authentic being, your spirit simply cannot be stopped.

I believe anything is possible when we put loving attention on ourselves and allow the alignment within us to click into place. All the parts of you that have been disconnected and ignored for years have been waiting for this very moment – for you to choose *you*. As a result of listening and committing to loving your body, you will receive miracles upon miracles from her. She will overflow her innate wisdom onto you by guiding you through life in the most magical ways. She will relax into a feeling of peace and contentment and will open up to more intimacy with self and others. You will feel free to be you, and to be seen in your unique and beautiful expressions of you. Your body has been waiting with eagerness to show you what's possible.

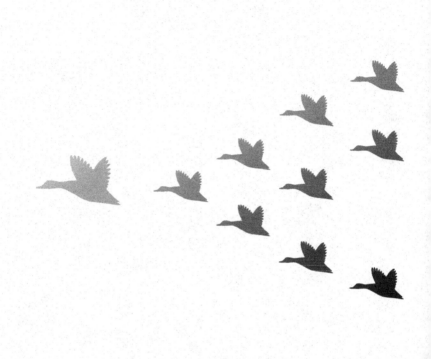

CHAPTER 2

MY FEAR FAT SUIT STORY

*"We delight in the beauty of the butterfly, but rarely admit the
changes it has gone through to achieve that beauty."*
— Maya Angelou

My story is one of self-forgiveness and of learning to love all
of me. I've dealt with a variety of traumas that added to
the creation of my fear fat suit but also, ultimately, my freedom.

WHO AM I?

My first experience of trauma was being caught between two
cultures – my Chinese immigrant household, where I felt the
safest, and the American culture, where no one looked or acted
like me.

From the time I went to preschool, I had already felt the
shame of not belonging. At five years old, I refused to go to
Chinese school because I had begun to feel the impact of
self-hatred brewing inside me. That's where my journey of having a splintered identity, and wishing I was different, began. I

hated being Chinese, and as I got closer to my teens, I became increasingly more embarrassed by my parents – mostly my mom because she was loud and bossy, had an accent and bad grammar, chewed with her mouth open, and basically had "immigrant behaviors" that appeared to be inferior compared to the American culture we lived in. Even though she was the valedictorian at the number one university in Taiwan and had a master's in biochemistry, it didn't matter. People treated her as if she was less than, and I followed suit by abandoning both her and my cultural heritage.

I grew up in a mostly black culture, and there was a part of me that wished that I was black. I just wanted to escape the feeling of being labeled all the things that Asians were made fun of for. From my young naive eyes, the black kids had it made because they were the popular kids. "Ching Chong" and other slurs were not an uncommon occurrence in my life.

By the time I went to high school, I changed my name to Stephanie because I hated my birth name. I hated myself. Each new school year, I would sneak into the classroom before class began and asked the teacher to call me 'Stephanie' during roll call. I hated when the other students called me Pong Ho or Ping Pong, so changing my name to Stephanie was my attempt at eliminating this abuse once and for all. I had hoped that by changing my name, I would be able to change how I felt too, but that wasn't how it turned out at all.

By the time I went to college, I changed my name again, this time to Chyna. I wanted to leave my trauma-filled high school years behind me and completely recreate myself. It was also an attempt, (albeit a warped one) at owning my Chinese identity. "Chyna" was a mask that allowed me to pretend to own my heritage, but it was just the other side of the self-hatred coin. I saw how the name Stephanie didn't change how people treated me in high school so I tried something different out of desperation. Little did I know, I was just running from the problem. It wasn't until I was twenty-five and went to China for the first time as an adult that I started to release the shame I held onto about being Chinese. I returned to my job and asked people to start calling me a name closer to my given name: Po. It was a beginning, and it meant something. As I began traveling down a long and winding path of self-love, I simultaneously started to fall in love with my name and many years later, was eventually was able to introduce myself fully as Po-Hong.

LOST AND NOT FOUND

As long as I can remember, I was always a highly sensitive and empathic child. I was the baby of the family and felt it was my responsibility to make sure my family felt connected. I saw myself as the hub of a wheel, the necessary element that needed to hold and keep my family together. So, when my parents divorced, when I was about eleven years old, I felt completely sideswiped, shocked, and alone. I was suddenly propelled into an unfathomable reality, and there was no communication about what was happening, or our feelings about any of it, because anything having to do with feelings was not a part of the culture my parents were raised in. This didn't mean my parents weren't loving, because they were, but they simply had no skills to offer me any support. Because of this, I experienced their divorce as a formative, traumatic event.

The family that I loved with my entire being was now in pieces. I now lived with my mom and new stepfather, Sifu. My dad moved to another home. My sixteen-year-old brother, whom I adored and had looked up to, left home under negative circumstances, and suddenly, I no longer felt close to him. Everything that I knew and loved was no more. I felt so scared and so alone and the grief felt insurmountable. I didn't understand what was happening inside of me, and I didn't have the language to express it. I just stayed silent, brewing in anguish, without support. There was an emptiness growing in me, and I wanted so badly to fill it. So I did just that; I unconsciously looked for love in all the wrong places.

At age eleven, when I first got my period, I was just about to enter into my teens and boom, my hormones and emotions kicked into full gear. Boys seemed like the answer to my prayers. Boys, I thought, could fill in what felt so empty and lonely in me. They gave me attention and I believed them when they told me what I wanted to hear. I was extremely naive and very shy. No one had explained sex to me. I was completely clueless about anything that had to do with boys, my body, or sex, and this left me in a vulnerable position.

One day, a seventeen-year-old boy named Thomas approached me in the park and his attention, words, and affection made me feel so special. His focus on me took my mind off of the pain of losing my family. He scheduled a hangout with me at his friend Mike's house and told me that Mike's mom would be home. But, when we arrived at Mike's house, Thomas casually said, "Oh his mom isn't home. She had to do something." Mike proceeded to bring Thomas and I down to the basement and then left us alone. I felt uneasy, and my body was screaming to get out of there, but I couldn't move. I was frozen in fear.

Thomas raped me. I was a twelve-year old child, a virgin, and there was bleeding, pain, and so much about the experience that stunned and traumatized me. I had neither the maturity or understanding to process any of it. I only noticed that Thomas seemed to have experienced some joy out of taking my virginity. To him, it was a badge of honor; now, according to him, he'd become a real man. I'm sure he told Mike all about it. I walked home quickly, in shock and confused about what had just happened. On the way home, I saw my dad, and I pretended to be okay. I casually told him I got my period and needed to clean up and even laughed it off.

The seed of shame and self-abandonment had been planted, and the next level of hiding began at exactly that moment. I felt dirty, but I didn't know why because I had no awareness that I had been raped. I didn't even know what rape was nor have the word 'rape' in my vocabulary. And since Thomas didn't physically hold me down, I thought something must be wrong with me. I was certain that because I felt bad, that this was my fault. I had allowed this. I was bad.

You see, even though I had no idea that my innocence and body had been violated, I had all of the symptoms a person who has been raped usually has. Almost like clockwork, my personality and appearance completely transformed. I went from a super shy girl to a loud, angry, and rebellious teen. I went from being at a healthy weight to gaining twenty pounds in less than a year. I started hanging with girls who drank alcohol and smoked weed to distract me from my pain.

I had my first real drink when I was thirteen. It was Bacardi 151 straight from the bottle. I recall the burning in my throat and stomach and the sense of calm that came over me. Numbness felt like heaven. I was so happy I had finally found something strong enough to numb all the pain I had been feeling for so long.

I was dying inside, so I attempted to die on the outside. I tried to commit suicide by taking a bottle of extra-strength Tylenol when I was thirteen years old. I wanted to escape so badly, to not exist, to just disappear and not feel anymore.

Fortunately, I woke up in the middle of that night with severe stomach pain and told my mom what happened, and she brought me to the hospital in a panic. I was then put in a halfway home for disturbed teens. My roommate had bulimia. I had to sleep there with all kinds of teens who I thought were way more troubled than me. Now looking back, I see I needed to be there. I was just as sick as the other kids there and I desperately needed help.

Unfortunately, I couldn't receive the help available there because I was mortified that the kids at my high school knew that I tried to kill myself. So, I convinced my therapist that I would never attempt suicide again. I told her that I had only done it for the attention, which was actually true and I realize now, surprisingly insightful for me to be aware of at that time in my life. I was crying for help but had no idea how to ask for it directly. I was released from the halfway home with the condition that we would begin family therapy, but when we tried it, it didn't really help the situation because I wasn't ready and my parents didn't know how to process their emotions. I hardly knew who I was. In hindsight, I believe that because I had experienced so much trauma without any tools to process it, or begin to heal from it, that I was completely shut down.

I continued to escalate with rebellious rage and simply did whatever I wanted: I snuck boys into my room, I got blackout drunk in the worst parts of Boston while hanging out with gang members and other guys I didn't know, I drove drunk. My mom had no idea what to do with me. I would yell curses at her and act out in the most awful ways imaginable while still being responsible working at a local bakery and going to school. I spiraled out of control and found myself in situations over the next three years where I was raped three more times, one of them being a gang rape. I had no regard for my body or my life because I lived outside of my body, completely disassociated from every aspect of my being. The innocent girl was left behind, and a new bad girl, 'who gives a crap?' version of myself emerged. A version that was hardened because it was the only way I could survive the pain, trauma, abuse, and self-hated. I felt like a disposable piece of meat that was only on this earth to be used for other people's needs and wants, and so I acted accordingly.

FEAR FAT SUIT

The rapes I experienced as a young person, on top of all the other accumulated pain from my self-identity issues and other traumas, implanted a deep-seated fear, rage, and shame in me, a shame that would take me decades to unravel and heal. The weight that I gained during that time became the physical manifestation of the emotional pain that I was trying to bury. I now call it my "fear fat suit."

Being overweight and chunky offered me a false sense of safety. It was a brilliant defense strategy for a young girl that didn't know what else to do to help herself. I didn't have the tools or internal resources to communicate my experience or ask for support.

Even though it was obvious that I was declining fast, no one knew how to help me. My parents came from a culture where kids didn't act out the way I did, so they had no idea how to support me and that made me feel even more alone.

As a consequence of these accumulated experiences, I lived in a state of victimhood for decades with the mask of an 'I don't care' attitude. I learned self-pity as a tool to get attention and manipulate others, and I used blame and shame to deflect responsibility. I became addicted to my drama, pain, and self-hate as a way to disconnect from my true self. My days were filled with mental spinning thoughts, judgments, and resentments leading to overwhelm and disconnection. No wonder why I smoked so much weed, binge drank alcohol, and indulged in emotional eating. I couldn't be with myself. I was imprisoned in a fear fat suit of my own making.

ROCK BOTTOM RADIANCE

When I was around twenty-seven years old, I was smoking weed all the time and drinking way too much. I had an addictive personality born of my sexual traumas. By this time, I had been numbing myself for many years with food, drugs, alcohol, and drama. Anything to escape. I don't know how I came across online gambling, but that became another source of escapism. And to be specific, I was most enthralled with blackjack, I played whenever I could and usually until all hours of the night. When I lost money, I wanted to play more so I could win it back. When I won money, I wanted to play more so I could win more. It was a disaster.

Ultimately, I ended up losing around thirty thousand dollars in a couple of weeks. Yes, you read that right: $30,000. I hit rock bottom yet again. I was already depressed, my lifestyle was a hot mess, and I had just gambled more of my life down the drain.

Miraculously, I made a choice to stop. I had a moment of clarity that I was never going to win my money back because the house always wins. I looked at the reality of the situation and saw how deep I had dug my hole, and I was afraid to go any deeper. I wasn't physically laid out on the ground, but emotionally I felt completely collapsed. Defeated. Done. I was already exhausted from fourteen years of addictive behaviors, depression, anxiety, PTSD, and all kinds of drama in relationships. And, now, this!

I will never forget the moment when, in my state of collapse, I had a vision. I saw myself in a dark tunnel. It was long, appearing almost endless. I was laying on the ground and wanting to give up. But then I lifted my head and looked up toward the end of the tunnel. I squinted my eyes and saw in the very far distance that there was light. It was the end of the tunnel. I could actually see an end in sight, even though it was just the tiniest glimmer, so tiny that it looked like a star in the sky.

It did, in fact, become my north star in that moment and for many moments in the next few years. I realized at that moment that that light represented hope and the possibility of happiness. Up until that point, I had been suffering from depression for so long that I didn't know if I would ever be happy. But that light reminded me that it was there, waiting for me as long as I moved toward it, because I believed it was possible for me.

So I started to crawl, at first like a baby, slowly and weakly, but it didn't matter. I was moving forward. I felt a desire igniting within me that came from my vision of getting to the light. I told myself that even if I had to crawl the entire time, I would do it. Then, what started happening was a miracle: I started crawling faster until I was able to stand. Then I could take small steps, and my speed started to increase. Years later, I made it out of that tunnel.

I reached the light, and it shined so brightly. Then I had an 'aha' moment, realizing that the light was me. I was reaching myself, my own radiance. After two decades of depression, I started to feel genuine happiness. I wasn't happy all the time. I was still struggling with sadness, anxiety, and loneliness, but I never thought I would feel happy at all. I was in awe and so truly proud of the work I had done. In spite of everything, I hadn't given up because my burning desire for happiness had fueled my path every step of the way. It was desire that had kept me going throughout all the moments I'd wanted to give up (and there were so many). Especially when my beloved mom suddenly passed a few months before my thirtieth birthday. I had such a hard time grieving her death because I didn't feel safe enough to feel all of the emotions inside of me. I used weed to numb out for a few years, but I always kept my eye on my vision with a kind of fierce determination despite any evidence to the contrary. I knew that happiness was possible for me if I just kept taking a step or two in that direction. Even in the darkest of moments, I held on to my hope and faith with my life.

BORN TO BE A SEEKER

As you can probably tell, even in the most stuck, dark, and unclear moments of my life, I have always been a seeker. I was raised by my dad who was my first spiritual teacher and continues to be my guide, my mom who was a fierce leader and truthteller, and my stepfather who was a grandmaster of Hung Gar Kung Fu, Qi Gong and Tai Chi as well as a Chinese herbal

25

medicine doctor. Their presence in my life has shaped the way I look at life as well as how I choose to live. Their own seeking gave me permission to seek too. They were courageous in trying new things, introspective, and service-oriented, and I too have found myself picking up those traits along the way.

In his younger years my Dad was a Jesuit Priest. Ultimately, he left the priesthood because he found the elders weren't practicing what they were preaching. His integrity could not abide with hypocrisy. In subsequent years he explored a variety of spiritual texts, philosophies and traditions, and eventually came to the Tao and settled there. He has been a consistent source of wisdom for me. The two of us have clocked in countless hours of conversations about yin and yang, the laws of energy, and nature in the back rooms of the laundromat my parents continued to own together, even though they were divorced. The laundromat was like my church, and apparently it was a sacred and meaningful space for others too because students would come to the laundromat to learn from his wisdom. His love is unconditional, and it continues to inspire me to be more graciously loving in my life. In fact, both his energy as well as his teachings will forever comprise the foundation of my work.

My mom was a biochemist turned business woman and activist and was always trying new things. She had a sharp mind and was always curious about new opportunities and was the reason why our family became middle-class. She was a boss lady, spoke her mind, didn't care what others thought of her, and had the most contagious laugh. She showed me what being a powerful woman and leader is. Her fire and courage continue to burn in me.

I remember taking kung fu in my stepfather's martial arts studio, which was in part of the same building as the laundromat. They were side by side and had a door that connected the two so you could easily go from the back room of the laundromat to the martial arts studio. The three of them were friends. Even in the midst of all my acting out and rage at my parents during my teens, having this space was a blessing because it was my home base.

Even though Sifu and I didn't communicate in words much, because we didn't speak the same language, he impacted me tremendously. He was my Chinese medicine doctor and inspired me to be a healer many years later. I recall a moment where he had a Qi Gong class and the students were lined up in a row with their eyes closed and after he took a moment to cultivate his energy, he proceeded to push their bodies without even touching them. That was my first time seeing the power of energy. Between the deep conversations I was having with my dad about energy and then actually seeing energy at work, my mind was blown.

Martial Arts was another blessing because it shaped the way I see things. The old school Kung Fu way of training was through observation so I had to notice every minute movement in order to learn the form. It taught me how to see the nuances in people and in situations that other people would skim over, and that has and continues to serve me well.

So as you can see, I was born to be a seeker. And as you'll see, I have gone through quite a healing adventure. This is how my path unfolded. In sharing my journey with you, I am not advocating for you to do the same; It's only to share more of me with you.

MY HEALING JOURNEY

Acupuncture school was my initiation into the healing world. I learned so much about myself, about the body, about energy, about my culture, about yin and yang. Helping others was the path to helping myself. As I became a clinician, I used my experience in treating my patients, to research and observe human nature and the mind-body connection. I was seeking answers and as a result was guided to plant medicine.

From the ages of thirty-seven to forty-three, I had gone through an intense journey of healing that took me down a rabbit hole of healing and discovery that was initiated by two ayahuasca retreats in 2013. Ayahuasca is a sacred plant medicine that is used in spiritual ceremonies among the indigenous people of the Amazon. It created an unseen and unspoken roadmap into my healing journey by guiding me with clear messages on what was next, like a magical adventure following the breadcrumbs.

It directed me to go to Michfest (Michigan Womyn's Music Festival), a place where thousands of womyn congregated in sisterhood on hundreds of acres of land which was called, "the land". It was held every August and on that particular year it was their thirty-eighth year! Imagine thousands of womyn camping out, going to workshops, eating, laughing, partying, showering, watching mind-blowing performances, and just being together. It was like a magical land where you could exhale and be you. And it was all created and built by womyn. Everyone was responsible to do volunteer shifts to keep this well-oiled machine going and it created an even richer sense of community. My heart was cracked open during my time there. I never felt so much community and generous overflowing love up until that point and with complete strangers! Making eye contact and greeting each other with "hello sister" or "sister my sister!" I could be naked in the woods and feel safe in my body. And seeing other womyn embodying their beautiful curves, shapes, and sizes inspired me to own and honor more of who I was at that time.

One day, I was in the womyn of color tent and was hanging out by the hammock with a group of womyn. One of them was looking through the program booklet and said, "there's a workshop called 'orgasmic meditation' in fifteen minutes. Anyone wanna go?" My body lit up and I was an immediate yes!

As soon as I heard the two women talk about how the practice allows you to let go of control and open to receiving, my body was a complete yes. This was exactly what I was desiring but didn't know how to get it.

As soon as I got back home to Brooklyn, I looked up the company that taught orgasmic meditation, OneTaste, and without blinking an eye, signed up for their ten-month coaching program that was held monthly in San Francisco. I didn't care about the commitment, money, or travel. My gut told me to go for it so I did.

I was completely triggered when I arrived at the first weekend. I had never been around that many white people in my life. Up until this point, most of my friends were black. But I could feel there was something powerful for me to receive, so I tried to keep an open mind. By the end of that weekend, I was sold on the practice even though I was still guarded. So much that I signed up for another program called Mastery that was to help you open up your sex. I continued to dive deep into their community and eventually took all of their programs over the next two years.

It was an intense healing environment and process, and I was connecting with people in an intimate and transparent way, which I hadn't ever done before. I was releasing so much of the sexual trauma and shame that was stored in my body for over two decades. I started to see myself with new eyes, practiced using my voice, and processing old emotions. Up until that point, I had been a complete control freak, disconnected from myself and others, sex was a disassociated experience and happened most often when I was drunk or high. But allowing myself to experiment in this sex-positive community gave me the opportunity to open up my sexuality in a new and profound way which began to rewire my trauma-filled conditioning.

During this time, I started to open back up to being sexually and emotionally intimate with men. I was with women only for eight years prior. It was a time of leaning into big edges, listening to my body, and discovering sensations in a body that had been numb for a lifetime.

Even though I had many rock bottoms up until this point, I had a unique and intense experience when I became one of the owners of OneTaste NYC. Even though I didn't agree with how the executives ran the company, it forced me to take a clear look at myself and my insidious victim mentality. The extreme nature of their culture pushed me to the edge and gave me an opportunity to really look at myself in the mirror. It motivated me to get sober emotionally and sober from alcohol and weed for a few years via the twelve-step program with a sponsor.

I remember that first day in an AA room clear as day. I had just returned from my second time at MichFest, which was their fortieth and final festival. But this time was unlike the last. I was so unhappy at OneTaste that I used MichFest as a way to escape with drugs. I took MDMA three times that week (I had only taken it once in my life before that) and five days after I returned home, I woke up in tears. I couldn't stop bawling my eyes out. I called out of work at OneTaste and got a massage and tried other self-care tools but the tears wouldn't stop. Then I got a text from a OneTaste peer and she suggested I go to an AA meeting without knowing what I had done at MichFest.

I had gone to other AA meetings before with the OneTaste community but this time was different. I cried throughout the meeting. I resonated with the stories and the shares. And at the end of the meeting, I was so in tears that I didn't notice that I was the only one in the middle of the room, surrounded by everyone standing in a circle holding hands. I immediately joined the circle and the love I received from perfect strangers cracked my heart open.

I ended up going to three meetings that day and decided that I was going to get sober because I felt significantly better by the evening. I felt the power of the rooms that day. So, I found a sponsor and she walked me through the 12 steps. And through her generous service and the steps, I saw with crystal clarity how fearful, resentful, manipulative, and selfish I had been most of my life, and that was a gift.

During this time, I started attending a new thought church called Celebration Spiritual Center. It felt like home because they spoke my spiritual language and taught what my dad and I always discussed; modalities like the law of attraction and nature herself being our best teacher. Being in this community brought a sense of lightness that I really needed at that time. The previous couple of years had been a powerful exploration of the shadowy parts of me, and it felt good to balance that out with the inspirational tone of their services. The songs, the teachings, the love touched my heart.

Then I found myself being guided intuitively to take a women's empowerment course taught by Regena Thomashauer, aka Mama Gena, an author and brilliant teacher of the power of the feminine. I heard of her through the OneTaste community but never had a desire to take her courses because I secretly judged her and her community without knowing anything about her. As I immersed myself in her teachings, I found myself nourished in a new and profound way through the healing balm of sisterhood and in the unique *"Sister Goddess"* community Mama Gena created. It was in this sacred container that I finally learned how to alchemize my rage and grief into a powerful force called "turn-on" by allowing myself to fully feel and embody my emotions. These tools were profound and life changing. "Turn-on" is an electrical current within you that arises when you are tapped into the deepest and widest range of your feminine being and emotions. As I practiced new tools and modalities, I began to shift from a suffering paradigm into a pleasure paradigm and learned how to embody all that lived within me.

THE CATALYST

Throughout those years, beginning at acupuncture school, I felt wave after wave of what I had begun to call awakenings. There was a moment, after a relationship ended in 2018 where I felt like I had come out of the "matrix". It was a dramatic breakup as was usually the case. I wanted to break my cycle of drama and heartbreak and this particular rupture gave me the motivation to change my ways. I felt ready to try something I hadn't tried before.

After breaking up with him, I felt an enormous weight of guilt, as if I was letting him down. I felt an addictive urge to rescue him, fix him, help him, even though he had done something extremely hurtful to me. It was my old friend, martyrdom, coming for a visit! My ego was in full-on torture mode and was trying to convince me that I was a horrible person. The guilt wouldn't stop. I was flogging myself. Then there was a moment of clarity that said, "You're making yourself responsible for his suffering, and it has nothing to do with you. He is responsible for himself."

My spirit told me to go to Celebration Spiritual Center and when I listened, I was introduced to a miraculous practice by Pastor Yolanda. After sharing with her what I was going through she suggested I try *The Work* by Byron Katie. With just four simple questions and a "turn around" prompt at the end, *The Work* is a profound meditative process that allows the truth to arise in you. *The Work* is done through challenging one thought or belief at a time, and as you question each one, your suffering dissipates organically.

Even though I intellectually knew that my thoughts and beliefs were holding me back, something clicked in my body, on a visceral level, when I did *The Work*. It was as if I'd gone from seeing life in splotches of color to experiencing my life in full technicolor. My vision was clearer, and my mind was so much calmer. Through *The Work*, I had a series of 'aha' moments that clicked in my body. I had two primary insights that completely shifted my life as I knew it. I realized that:

- I was addicted to suffering and drama because it was what I was used to and comfortable with, which meant that I was *choosing* to suffer.
- If it was true that this was a choice, then I had the power to choose something else!

Guilt was the perfect co-conspirator in helping me heal because every time I felt it, I knew it was a chance for me to feel the deeper emotions from my past that lived underneath it. It was a blessing in disguise that my ex was persistent in trying to win me back with passive-aggressive attempts, trying to make me feel bad. There are no accidents. He mirrored exactly what I needed to heal. Instead of letting my initial feelings of seeing him as a jerk or blaming him for acting like a child, I used those opportunities to practice my boundaries. I kept saying no with firmness and love. Each time, the guilt would decrease, and my self-compassion increased. I felt stronger in myself.

I also added self-forgiveness into the mix. Instead of putting attention on forgiving him, I focused on forgiving myself for all the ways I participated in the unhealthy dynamic between us. This didn't mean that I didn't hold him accountable for the parts that he played. It means that I held myself accountable for the parts *I* played. This required me to rise up in self-compassion in a way I never had up until that point in my life. This was a radical departure from the way I was used to operating.

As a result of months of intense deep diving belief work, I was able to let go of my root belief that I am responsible for everyone's well-being and suffering, and from there, the beliefs that branched off of that one root belief began to dissipate on their own. This then allowed me to naturally redirect the attention and energy I always had spent on others, onto myself and release my physical weight with more ease and pleasure. Something I had never been able to do up until that point.

RELEASING THE WEIGHT

When you picked up this book, you may have thought this was a typical dieting book. Surprise! It's definitely not. Instead, I aim to show you how being intuitively led from a transformed belief system, while connecting with how you feel in your body, mind, spirit, and soul can help you to effortlessly release weight as well as bring in so much joy and fulfillment.

It's important to note that I was falling in love with myself *before* I lost the weight and continued to love myself more as the journey continued. This wasn't about releasing the weight and then loving myself. It doesn't work that way. Many people try it in that order, and they either gain the weight back because they don't feel comfortable in their new body or they feel bad on the inside even though they have a new body.

My physical lifestyle before releasing my martyr story was an inactive one filled with unconscious eating habits. I pretty much never exercised. Looking back at my life spanning over four decades, in total I had three shortish spurts where I exercised, of approximately three years in all: When I was in my teens, I took my stepfather's Kung Fu class for less than a year. When I was twenty-nine years old, I was swimming regularly for less than a year. When I was forty-one, I took boot camp for about a year. I hated walking anywhere. I even drove to work in NYC because I didn't want to take the train or walk. Plus, I felt safer in my car. Again, more hiding.

Emotional eating began when I was a child. Food was one of my security blankets. I loved food. I would always clean my plate, and I ate pretty much anything. There's a joke with one of my oldest friends that her father loved me so much because I would always eat all of his food, clean the plate, and go for seconds. I ate unconsciously. Just stuffing food in my mouth whenever I wanted without thinking about it.

But when I finally released my martyr story, I felt my body whispering to me that it was time to do the physical work. Now I was able to hear what my body was communicating with me every step of the way. I did things that I never thought I wanted to do like jogging, but since my body told me to, I did it. My body told me to do mirror work and intermittent fasting, and so I did those too. My body even told me to grow out my bangs. So I did it! As I continued to follow the wisdom of my body, I continued to fall in love with myself and the different aspects of me which I had judged so fiercely in the past. And then the weight just came off because my body and I became the best of friends. The trust was established.

I incorporated a goal-setting system which kept me account-able to myself. I also created a community of women who also wanted to release their physical and emotional weight because I knew how important it is to have a community for witnessing, fun and added accountability on the journey. Before I knew it, I lost forty pounds and fifteen percent body fat in about five months, and I felt strong, alive, and confident!

Healing starts from the inside first. Releasing weight is something that anyone can force themselves to do if there's enough willpower, but willpower only lasts so long. I am more interested in what's sustainable and what feels good. That is an authentic, living, practice of self-love.

THE OTHER SIDE

I'm on the other side of my traumas now because I did the work that was being asked of me. The outcome is that I have so much gratitude for all of it – my family splitting up, my rapists, the suicide attempt, all the pain. If it weren't for my traumas, I wouldn't be able to talk to you right now about releasing *your* body armor. I wouldn't be able to empathize with so many people and ultimately become a healer, teacher, and author. I wouldn't have been able to explore my darkness as deeply as I have.

I believe that the brightness of my light is in direct correlation to the depths of the darkness that I have injected love into. The more I was able to hold space for my darkness with love and bring it into the light, the more I was able to feel that light within me. We all have a history of pain, but when it stays hidden, there is no way to love on it. There is no way to transmute it. The light needs to come out. It needs to shine. You need to shine! I believe this process of alchemy is the only way to touch, taste, and embody the light that is living in you.

I can now share the story of what's possible when you move *through* it, not around it. It opens up universes of possibilities that are beyond your wildest imagination. I'm not only referring to the abundance that you can manifest in your life in the forms of financial wealth, community, success, or having the body of your dreams. I'm mostly referring to peace of mind, the feeling of happiness and connection within you. That's the gift of taking this life adventure into your own hands.

I am writing this book from a place of honoring my darkness and my light and *all* of the participants in my life, whether they appeared to be "good" or "bad." They all led me to where I am at this moment.

THE
FOUNDATION

CHAPTER 3

INSIDE OUT

"The part can never be well unless the whole is well."
— Plato

The process I'm going to take you through is about revealing who you are underneath all of the layers of shame, pain, and fear that you have been holding on to. It's about remembering that you are whole and that you don't need to be fixed. You may need to thaw the layers of protection that you have been built around yourself, but you were born whole and complete and you will always remain that way no matter what.

From what I've observed, many brilliant women, such as yourself, are chasing the dragon of healing and hoping that they will come out on the other side of the course fixed, and as a result, are coming up feeling even more broken when that doesn't happen. You can go to the best seminars, have the most profound plant medicine ceremonial experiences, read all the self-help books, be mentored by brilliant mentors, and understand all of the deepest philosophies but that doesn't guarantee you will create long lasting freedom in your life. There is no magic pill. You have to do the work in all the realms – the emotional, mental, and physical. There's no way around it.

From my observation, women are using their intelligence to try to "figure it out" or "fix" their problems once and for all. From my experience, this will never work because intelligence can only get you so far. Intelligence allows us to grasp an idea and learn about important philosophies or practices. But in order to create fully integrated and sustainable shifts, meditative states of consciousness need to be cultivated, inhabited, and fully lived inside the body. I'm not just talking about sitting meditation, which is crucial in order to do this work, but I'm referring to being connected to your inner landscape of emotions, thoughts, and sensations as you live each moment of your life.

The process I teach is based off of yin and yang and entry points. It's a process of taking full advantage of what's activated for you in your life and using these activations to do the excavation work that your spirit is yearning for. To be present within these highly charged moments, with integrity, can shift everything. As you practice holding space for the entire spectrum of whatever is arising, you will begin to be led down a path meant for you. Sometimes this is called being in a 'flow state' or working with the wisdom of the Tao.

YIN AND YANG

As an acupuncturist, I always treat the root cause. The symptoms are treated as well, but the priority is the catalyst for the imbalance. It's no accident that my dad is a Taoist spiritual teacher as Taoism is the foundation of acupuncture.

Taoism is based on nature and is expressed through the relational dynamics of yin and yang and how they flow and interact together. They are opposite yet complementary energies.

Yin is the feminine and represents the fluids (like blood), the deeper internal aspects of self, and the darker, slower, more intuitive, receptive, accepting, and subtle aspects of self and life.

Yang is the masculine and represents the qi (energy), the outer aspects of self, where the light hits, and the structured, dominant, and moving aspects of self and life.

Taoism is rooted in nature and the organic flow between the yin and yang. In order to understand how to receive the transmission of my teachings, it's crucial to understand the nature of yin and yang and their relationship to each other.

When you look at the yin and yang image, you see that the black is yin and the white is yang, and they have a dot in the middle of each with the opposite color.

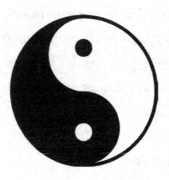

This symbol conveys the relationship between the two. That they are not separate from each other. They are actually interconnected, and the movement of one directly affects the movement of the other. They are two energies that are one, and are very much alive. They fluctuate and change just like nature. The knowledge and integration of this ancient wisdom will allow you to connect to your flow because yin and yang are in constant flow.

You can see this dynamic everywhere you look. Everything is made up of a mix of the two. Each person, each project, each relationship. And within each person, or thing, lies another layer of yin and yang. You can break anything down to its yin or yang aspect. And this information is so vital as you move through this process because it will help you to identify exactly where you are in the balance of the two.

The beautiful thing about the Tao is that there's an innate sense of compassion because there are no expectations of what is supposed to be or not be.

You will find that what I teach is a combination of internal (yin) and external (yang) work as well as fluid (yin) and structured (yang) work. Also, in line with this philosophy, you will find that there is a balance of compassion (yin) and commitment (yang) in the approaches. It's all about balance and how each element flows and dances with the other. Not one piece is isolated from another. They are one and interact with each other in a symbiotic way and this is what creates a sense of peace and flow into your life.

ENTRY POINTS

It's so interesting how human beings are usually motivated to make significant changes in their life by desperation, not inspiration. Life will happen, and unforeseen life events will unfold that will cause you immense pain. That's part of being human. No one is immune to "negative" experiences, devastation or loss, no matter how much we try to protect ourselves, but we can use them for our benefit.

Being a child of immigrant parents, I was given the gift of resourcefulness. Inherently, I hate to waste. I don't like to waste food, money, or good old-fashioned pain. My dad taught me many years ago that challenges are gifts from the Universe. Are you going to toss it aside or are you going to open up that gift and see what's inside waiting for you?

That always stayed with me, and since then, I always make sure to take advantage of life's challenges and use them to propel me to the next level of my growth. It's like an emotional leveraging system. We can use these little or big life events as stepping-stones if we allow ourselves to walk through the portal, versus around it.

This is where my creation of the entry point process was born. When we choose to allow our pain or discomfort to be an entry point into our healing, the Universe works with us as a co-creator and guides us in miraculous ways. It's being resourceful to the next level – tapping into the bounties of the unseen world.

This is an advanced form of gratitude practice and as I continued to practice it, I found myself going deeper into revealing more of who I am. What I found was more love. That's why I always say that heartbreak allows more love into your life because it gives you an opportunity to feel and uncover parts of you that may have been dormant for years, or even decades,

There are three entry points: emotional, mental and physical. Within each realm lies an entry point that can be activated by emotions, thoughts, and sensations respectively. If an entry point is activated, there is an opportunity to go deeper within yourself and discover the parts of yourself that have been suppressed. Whenever something vital is suppressed, flow is blocked and you are running aspects of your life from an unconscious place. This process is the guts of the work I teach. It's meditative, alchemical, and transformative. When you do the work in all three realms, energetic flow is a natural byproduct.

ALCHEMY

I have heard many stories of people releasing their weight and then gaining it back because they bypassed the self-love work. It happens all the time. Bypassing is an epidemic in our culture. It basically means that you're not willing to be with yourself exactly where you are because it is too uncomfortable to be present with the discomfort of your emotions, thoughts, or sensations. So you choose to bypass, which ultimately means that you are numbing.

Alchemy is the way beyond this. Walking through the portals that open when entry points are activated is an alchemical process. It's the process of revealing the shadows into the light and shows you how to create space in your life, and within yourself, so you can be fully present. Because where presence is, love is. It takes a lot of courage to be present with the parts of you that have been ignored, pushed down, and abandoned. It will probably be one of the most courageous things you'll ever have to do, but the upside to those acts of bravely investing in loving yourself will pay you back in self-love dividends which will multiply exponentially over time.

RECEIVING ALL THE BENEFITS

This book is divided into four sections. The Foundation, The Yin Portal, The Yang Portal, and The Other Side. The first section is the preparation and foundation needed before entering into the healing portal. The second section is the portal where you'll learn how to be a conscious practitioner and alchemize your activated entry points. The third section is about turning on your body, self-care, creating new habits, and goal setting. And the fourth section is about you emerging from the portal and into a lifetime of radiance and sustainable flow.

The best way to make the most of this book is to open up your mind and heart while reading. This is an alchemical process which means it requires willingness to see and do things differently. I invite you to see this as a journey where miracles abound and to see me as guide into new and unfamiliar territories. I will show you places that you may never have explored so courage is required on this trip. Please allow my words to travel into the deepest parts of your body, mind, heart, and spirit. Don't use your intellectual mind to understand or figure anything out. Receive the deeper messages that I am sharing with you by being present with the energy of my transmission.

After you read each chapter, sit and be still with your eyes closed for a few minutes and let that chapter's messages integrate into your system by being present with your breath.

You will notice that I recommend after each ritual to take a moment to thank yourself, source energy (or whatever you consider your higher power), your ancestors, and loved ones on the other side. Acknowledging your gratitude for those who are energetically holding you, loving you, and guiding you is a powerful way to close a ritual.

I invite you to take each chapter at your own pace and notice when you are resisting, when you're going too fast, and when you're not being kind to yourself.

You may want to keep a journal handy just in case you have an 'aha' that arises or a question that you want to explore so you can write it down as a reminder for later.

I suggest that you read the chapters in order, as one builds on top of the next. Just imagine each chapter as a stepping-stone. But after you read the book, you will practice blending all the steps together as a way of life.

You will notice that I use the phrase *releasing* weight instead of *losing* weight. I find that releasing weight feels more active and accountable while losing weight sounds more passive and less empowering. When you release something you are choosing to let it go. When you lose something, you can't find it and are looking to get it back.

And lastly, I cannot stress enough that my system for releasing weight is *not* about getting skinny. Our culture has conditioned us to think we need to look a certain way in order to meet society's patriarchal and racist standards of beauty. These messages will not serve your emerging magnificence and radiance. I want to offer you a journey that is meant for you to connect with what feels good to *you* and to truly live joyfully and peacefully inside of *your* body after many years of living outside of it. As you travel along this journey and work with the rituals and experiments I suggest, your goals may shift dramatically. Perhaps you think you want to release forty pounds, but once you release twenty pounds and you feel fantastic and no longer desire to release a fraction of a pound more. Or perhaps you fall in love with your body exactly as it is right now. Regardless of what your goal is, my desire is to assist you in cultivating a healthy and pleasurable life and a sustainable, delicious relationship with your body. I want to introduce you to powerful practices that will help you plug into the boundless potential of energy that is available to you and to every person living on the planet.

RIPPLE EFFECTS OF LOVE

One of my biggest desires is to create ripple effects of healing and love throughout the world. I have seen so many people attempt to make changes in the world, but they are giving from a place of empty and exhausted, obligation and fear, or over-whelm and resentment. None of these work. They may affect surface changes temporarily, but they're not sustainable over a lifetime. My mission is to remind people that changing the world must start from inside of each individual.

You see, the micro and macro levels are identical. What's happening on the inside is happening on the outside and vice versa. If we all prioritized our healing and connection with source energy, a higher power, the universe (or whatever term feels right for you) then there would be a natural overflow of goodness rippling throughout the world. The keyword here is *natural.* There is a more lasting and impactful change in our culture when it is organic and arising from an authentic con-nection to love. When we truly love ourselves, all of our inter-actions shift. We interact with strangers, our loved ones, our peers, and our communities in a much more profound and human way. Practicing kindness to ourselves *naturally* over-flows onto others, and that kindness continues to ripple from one person to the next. This is a fundamental law of energy and this is the way we can change the world. Seriously, think about it! Imagine, if you will, a massive ripple effect of love coming from each person's love for themselves, spreading outward.

The problem is that our culture is obsessed with external conditions, and as a result, we've become robots that have been brainwashed and conditioned by what generations of our ancestors have passed down and what society has taught us. We have taken on lies upon lies and received them as if they were

Truth with a capital T. Those lies will have you believe that you are not lovable, desirable, or worthy or that you have to look a certain way in order to deserve love. Those lies tell you that if you aren't "perfect" or don't do things "perfectly", you are not enough. We will address how to shift your stories and limiting beliefs, but first, you must be willing to see that you truly have been hypnotized. We all, without ever intending to do so, have drunk the proverbial Kool-Aid.

I want you to understand that loving your body is key to loving yourself. Your body is the vessel you were born into, and this is the vessel you will die in. There's no changing that. You might as well love your flesh and enjoy it. Because, think about it, if you don't love your body, then you have declared war on yourself. Loving all the perfectly imperfect human parts of us is vital to our feeling whole, alive, and complete.

CHAPTER 4

MEET YOUR NEW
BEST FRIEND

"Courage is the most important of all the virtues because without
courage you can't practice any other virtue consistently."
— Maya Angelou

INTO THE TUNNEL RITUAL

T*he journey into the portal begins with igniting your internal engine. Imagine you are in a car and you've parked in front of a secret tunnel. That tunnel represents a healing portal and you are about to drive through it. The first thing you must do is make sure your car is ready to go with a full tank of gas. Imagine you've made sure that your oil is changed and your tires are balanced. Now, imagine turning on the car with a special golden key and igniting your engine.*

Notice how this creates a spark that gets the juices flowing and warmed up. Your engine is humming.

Check you mirrors and, while you're at it, give yourself a wink.

Now, imagine a life in which, much like driving this imaginary car, you take your power back and put your attention on the only thing you can control: You. Are you ready? Make sure you've buckled your seatbelt because taking responsibility for your vehicle (your life) takes courage!

OWN YOUR DESIRES

In order to commit to this new adventure, there needs to be a desire that backs it up. How can you commit to something that has no anchor or passion connected to a bigger vision? You can't. It has to come from feeling what it is you truly desire in your life.

When we allow ourselves to feel our desires in our body and spirit, there's a deep knowledge that anything is possible. The more specific you can get with your desires the better. Use all of your senses. Let yourself get giddy at the thought of this vision that you see in your mind's eye. Feel how real it is and that knowing will create a frequency of vibration that will co-create with the Universe - you will receive all the support and resources you need. That person you see in your vision, is living in you right now. Many people are trying to create from an intellectual place and that will only take you so far. You must bring all of your senses on board for miracles to happen.

"Desires are the interface between you and that which is greater than you. Desires are where creation begins."
—Regena Thomashauer aka "Mama Gena"

DESIRE RITUAL

Sit in a quiet and private space and close your eyes and take three deep breaths. Feel your breath move through your body. Allow yourself to deeply inhabit your body.

From this place of embodiment, try to visualize in your minds-eye how you desire to feel in your body as well as in your life. Let yourself explore how your life would be if you release your physical and emotional weight.

Where are you? What are you doing? What are you wearing? How does it feel?

Let this imagery play out like a movie trailer. This is your life. This is you. Feel the realness of this in your body. Get excited. Feel the goodness.

Explore for a few minutes and when you feel complete, take three full breaths and then slowly open your eyes. Thank yourself, your higher power, and your loved ones on the other side for holding you through this experience.

Finally, journal about what you saw and experienced. Solidify it in your body through the act of writing.

If you want to take it one step further, create a vision board of what you saw and felt. Have fun with it! Once you're done keep in a familiar place so it can continue to inspire you.

COURAGE

Courage comes from a place of being completely and utterly loyal to yourself. It requires becoming selfish in the most positive life-affirming way, meaning that you give to yourself without taking anything away from anyone else. What makes you happy? What brings you peace? What feels pleasurable to you?

Courage is about embodying a warrior spirit of self-love. You have to prioritize how you feel before anything else, including your children, your partner(s), your work, your anything. Until you devote yourself *to* yourself you will be locked in a cycle of caretaking and resentment. If you are not putting yourself first, you will drain your energy consistently over time and will likely feel unclear, uninspired, and unhappy. You will find yourself living your life for others and wondering what happened to all the time that passed and why it is that your life looks and feels the same as it did five, ten, or even twenty years ago.

It also takes courage to meet yourself exactly where you are. Whether your mind is having obsessive thoughts or you are angry and full of rage, the ability to be present in those spots is a huge act of courage. Trying new things takes courage too. The willingness to read this book and to try some of the rituals are acts of bravery. When I shared the portal entry ritual with one of my clients she was terrified. She literally thought she was going to go into a pit of darkness and would never come out. Agreeing to try it, despite her fears, took courage.

It takes courage to be radically honest with yourself and to love yourself unconditionally. It takes courage to create a deeply intimate relationship with yourself and with source energy. It takes unbelievable courage to trust the process.

Every time I have expanded in my life, whether in career, money, sex, love, or relationships, the expansion happened when I took a step, jump, or leap of faith. I listened to my intuition and then took action. I have taken many big leaps of faith in my life, and I'm sure lots of people have questioned my sanity, but I always knew that the most important thing for me was to follow my internal guidance system. In order to follow this deeper knowledge, you truly must have the courage of a warrior. And in order for you to hear this intuition, you must trust the process and have faith that all will be revealed in due time.

PLEASURE RESEARCHER

I first heard this term in Mama Gena's Mastery program, and it struck me right away because I adore the idea of viewing life as a one big 'research' project. I've researched sex, boundaries, new ways of giving and receiving, being a victim, and more healing modalities than I can count. I've researched different relationship styles, careers, different places to live, but not once did I consider researching pleasure! Deciding to become a pleasure researcher was a radical step for me because the patriarchy has conditioned women to choose suffering and to believe that it is her lot in life. When a woman prioritizes pleasure, when she decides to investigate what exactly lights her up instead of numbs her out, she puts herself in the driver's seat and is on her way to a much more fulfilling life. Becoming a pleasure researcher is not only a personal act of courage but is also a brave, political act.

When I began my weight releasing process, I made sure to absolutely frame it as a pleasure research project. Why? Because in the past, trying to release weight was always miserable and frustrating, and this time I was determined to find joy in connecting with my body. When I injected "turn-on" and "pleasure" into the mix, everything shifted. Do you know what gives you pleasure? If not, I suggest you do some research.

By the way, real pleasure is not just doing whatever you want to do, whenever you want to do it. It's not eating all your kids' Halloween candy either.

I don't know about you, but I'm a curious person and love exploring and experimenting. When you choose to make this weight releasing process a research project, the entire game flips because it's not so serious. It's an experiment.

So put on your pleasure researcher hat, your lab coat, or whatever sounds fun to you and let's dive in a bit more.

PLEASURE RESEARCH RITUAL

Take out a pen and paper and write down all the things that bring you pleasure, from the itty-bitty things to the mouth-watering things.

Then write down all the items on your to do list that you dread, that make you want to procrastinate or pull your hair out.

Before you do a task, first do one pleasurable thing and get the joy factor up and the electricity in your body flowing.

For example, I used to hate doing my taxes until I paired it with dance breaks. I would take a dance break before I started and every twenty minutes or every time I felt my energy decrease or felt foggy or irritated.

MAKING YOURSELF # 1

Right out of the gate, in order to do this alchemical self-loving work, you must choose yourself first. There is no other way around it. You must make a commitment to your pleasure and peace. This means you will need to make hard decisions about downsizing and simplifying your life. It means that you will have to say 'no' to projects, friends and family, and experiences that you are not saying 'hell yes' to. It means that you will see your energy, time, and space as hot commodities and that these are not up for bargaining. No way!

Making this commitment is the key to creating the change you will require when it comes to releasing weight.

The way you start to choose you is by slowing down in your life and pausing to ask yourself what you really want to prioritize and cutting out the rest. Only keeping the essential things, the quality things. And letting go of what's not working in your life as well as not adding unnecessary stress. Let go of the clutter in your mind, space, and life. Release those distractions so you can have the space to choose something different. Pick wisely by feeling into what is the most important things to you. And then observe how having that space impacts your life.

MARIE KONDO THAT SH*T RITUAL

Take a birdseye view of your life. What parts of your life feel spacious and what parts of your life feel tight? Here's some common areas where people clutter their life:

- *Does your home feel cluttered?*
- *Do you have a gazillion to-do's on your list?*
- *Do you have events on your calendar that you don't feel excited about?*
- *Do you bring work home with you or you stay at work late all the time?*

Pick one of these areas that feels the most exciting or vital to declutter. Begin to consciously release what does not "spark joy" as Marie Kondo would say, and the ones that are not prioritizes.

Release with gratitude and feel the spaciousness that has been created.

Finally, take a moment to thank yourself for this brave act of letting go.

When you commit to yourself, you are also saying 'yes' to the process. But how do you commit to the process if it's something that you've already tried over and over again and feel you've failed at? You change your mindset and decide to fall in love with the process itself. You *choose* to get turned on by it so much that your journey becomes an exciting adventure, a new passion. You feel so turned on about what you're desiring to create in your life that you can't not love the journey, even when it's messy and challenging.

I encourage you to surrender to this process that I'm laying out for you in this book. I'm pretty sure that it's completely different than any other weight releasing process you've ever tried before. This is not a one and done deal. It's a life's work that will continue because it's not only about releasing the weight, it's about creating an intimate relationship with yourself.

MAKING THE CHOICE

Do you choose you first? This is the most important question in this book and it's the question that I had to answer for myself when I was at a crossroads. I looked in front of me and I saw the fork in the road. The left path was the one I had been on endless amount of times, my entire life. I saw all of my failures and suffering and it was filled with bad energy. Then I looked to the right and I saw another path that I had never been on. Completely new territory with many question marks but there was an air of possibilities. I knew that I had to make this radical choice of prioritizing me, no matter what, in order for my life to shift in the ways I wanted. So I chose the path on the right. What will you choose?

CROSSROADS RITUAL

Sit in a quiet and private space. Close your eyes and get in your body by taking a few deep breaths.

Picture a crossroads in the path and you're standing right there at the fork.

Visualize what the two different path looks like. Are there trees around? Is it bare? What's in the distance? Take a moment to really take it in.

And one at a time, take each one in. First, put your attention on the left path. The path that you have taken already. Take as much time as you need to see and feel what comes up when you put your attention on it. Any images, words, feelings, sensations arise? And when you feel complete, put your attention on the right path and do the same thing. Take your time and be with the experience.

When you're finished taking in the energy of each one, put your attention on both paths and compare the energies and scenery. What are the differences? How do they feel in comparison to each other?

With your eyes still closed, ask yourself, "which path do I choose?" And only with a "left" or "right" answer, allow your inner voice to answer. It's usually the first answer that arises and it feels real and good in your body. Your mind may want to enter and try to convince you of things, but stay with what feels right in your body.

When you receive your answer, take a few deeps breaths and open your eyes.

Lastly, take a moment to thank yourself, your higher power, and your loved ones on the other side for holding space for you in this exploration.

If you chose the right path, congratulations! Continue on to the next chapter.

If you chose the left path, congratulations! You will stay here until you are able to make this commitment to yourself. Knowing that you are resistant to prioritizing yourself is actually a good thing. Clarity is gold. Perhaps before this meditation, you thought you were ready to commit but now you're seeing you're not. This is good because you are being radically honest with yourself, whereas before you were trying to convince yourself or trying force yourself into something that wasn't right for you in that moment.

So instead of going into judgement or a self-analyzing mindset, I urge you to do another ritual that will support you in committing to this process.

LEFT PATH RITUAL

Journal for ten minutes about why you choose the left path. Be open and transparent about what's holding you back. Really feel into the blockages. Give yourself permission to explore all of the reasons and beliefs that are keeping you from choosing you first. Notice when you are making excuses for why you can't prioritize yourself. Dump all of your resistances onto the paper. Write down everything you can think of that is holding you back.

When you feel complete, do the Desire Ritual at the beginning of this chapter once more. Reconnect with your desire for wanting to shed your body armor. Feel that desire in your body. And when you're ready, do the Crossroads Ritual again.

You can do them back to back or the next day. You don't want to overload your system but you also don't want to bury this important decision under the rug. This process will give you even more clarity and perhaps the desire to try something new.

Each time you complete a ritual, take a moment to thank your-self, your higher power, and your loved ones on the other side for holding space for you in this pivotal moment in your life.

You may be thinking, why are you being so tough? And the answer is, because I love you. My job is to set you up to win. And in order for you to do that, you must be grounded in making you and your joy your number one priority. Until you commit, the rest of the other steps will be full of resistance and it will be next to impossible to do the subsequent work. This process isn't about forcing you to do something that you don't want to do. It's about your desire being so strong and clear that you feel the pull to do the work.

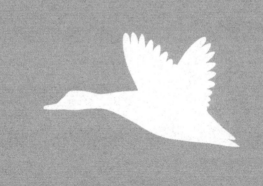

THE YIN PORTAL

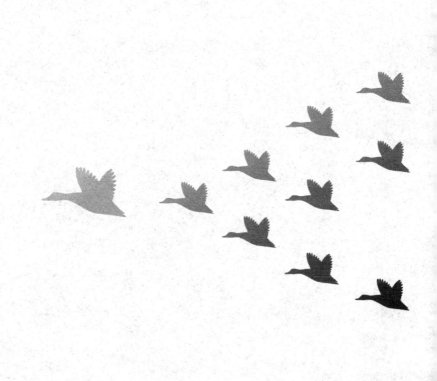

CHAPTER 5

LEARNING TO BE WITH YOURSELF

"The wound is the place where the Light enters you."
—Rumi

ENTRY POINTS

Imagine you're a detective and you are hot on the trail of solving a mystery that you were hired for. You have been finding clues and are on the hunt to see where they lead. That is what an entry point is. A clue that leads you into a spot that wants attention. They give you an opportunity to be present with what is wanting to arise from within you.

Entry points are activated all the time in these three realms: emotional (emotions), mental (thoughts), and physical (sensations). When they're activated, the typical responses range from numbing to losing control but you're going to use entry points to your benefit and as an opportunity to peel layers off and go deeper within yourself. So, put on your detective hat and get ready to explore!

They are gold nuggets but sadly they are usually tossed aside as if they are the culprit when in fact they're really the unsung heroes. If we see them for what they are, the perfect portals for alchemizing, we would be able to take our power back. This is about being resourceful and using these gifts by transmuting the once negatively charged energy into love, which is power. Since everything carries energy, when you transmute these potent entry point activations, your energy will increase. The "negative" activations carry intense energy just waiting to be alchemized.

It's one thing to be able to connect with the emotional, mental, and physical realms independently; it's a whole other thing when you are connecting with all of them simultaneously. It's common for people to avoid at least one realm and put most of their energy on the one(s) they are well versed in or feel more comfortable with. Also, it's quite possible that if you are focusing on a comfort-zone realm, you may end up spinning your wheels by avoiding the work that could have the most impact.

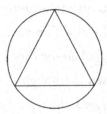

For example, when an emotion arises, you may think that you are feeling your emotions but really you are, in your mind, perseverating on a negative storyline thereby blocking the emotion underneath which is practically begging to be felt.

As you can see in the image, the circle only connects if you're doing the internal work in *each* entry point. The circle indicates flow, which is the balance of yin and yang and being so in tune with the moment that you are able to feel and trust your internal guiding system. It's living from a place of surrendering to your intuition and receiving the abundance that comes from that openness. You feel the divine within you, guiding you, right in the midst of everything that is happening in your world.

Now imagine within each activated entry point is a spiraling portal opening up. You have the choice to walk through it or you can continue to avoid it. This is the time to connect with your courage and make a decision to honor your deepest truths that have not yet been explored but desperately want to be.

The process I share below is how you walk through these portals and the following three chapters breakdown the process individually for each realm.

It's important to note that any activation is potent and worthy of attention. It could be micro moments throughout the day like a stranger looking at you in a certain way, to more monumental experiences like death. They all deserve respect. And in my experience, I find the "smaller" activations to be just as powerful because they are happening all the time. Imagine sweeping all of those juicy opportunities under the rug? Not this non-wasting first generation Chinese woman!

The practices I teach are meant to begin in a safe, quiet, and private container so you can cultivate your ability to hold space for yourself with no extra distractions. But ultimately, the practice is intended to touch every area of your life, when the moments arise: waking up in the morning, while in a conversation, walking to the train station, hanging out with friends, walking your dog, being on the phone, fighting with your partner, getting pissed at work, and/or grieving death.

The first order of business, before diving into the portal, is to get you into the practice of meditating.

SITTING MEDITATION

One of the best ways to travel through the portal and cultivate a connection to the yin and yang flow is meditation.

Meditation is so powerful because you receive so much in just one practice. You cultivate compassion, learn how to be with yourself, practice concentration, get to know yourself intimately, connect with your senses, heal your body through deep relaxation, expand your awareness, and develop the mindset of a conscious practitioner.

It took me many years to discover what an actual practitioner is, even though I had been one all my life. We all are practitioners because we are all practicing something all the time, whether it's conscious or subconscious. But when you are a conscious practitioner, you are able to see what's happening in your thoughts and behaviors closer to real-time or in real-time and make conscious loving choices based off of that awareness.

For the majority of my life, I was practicing beating up on myself, blaming and shaming myself and others, and overall being a control freak. Then, after taking self-development courses and learning about the power of our intention and attention, I saw that being a conscious practitioner is what it all comes down to.

Meditation also restores the body. Your body must be relaxed in order for the cellular aspects of the body to recover as well as the emotional body to release what it has been gripped onto. Meditation can help with sleep issues, releasing diseases, reducing anxiety and depression, and any physical ailment that has been caused by stress, which, in my clinical experience, is the majority of issues. There have also been endless research studies that have confirmed the role stress plays in creating disease in the body.

Meditation helps you become more attuned to what's happening inside you. Your mindfulness and consciousness naturally open and you're able to see and feel things that you couldn't before. I remember a time I had been struggling to meditate regularly for years, but once I committed to the practice, my entire life shifted. Not surprisingly, I had hit a bottom and that's when I decided to commit to my meditation process. I felt more grounded and was more kind to and patient with myself. Clarity started to replace my fogginess and confusion. I could connect with the idea of progress, not perfection, in my actual day-to-day life. Years later, my meditation practice has expanded and impacts me in even more profound ways. I now feel the divine love and power, that is available to all, living within me.

Whether you already meditate or not, I highly recommend reading or listening to *Stress Less, Accomplish More* by Emily Fletcher. It's a great book for beginners and non-beginners because it teaches a meditation technique that is incredibly simple and inspires you to commit to the practice. For first-time meditators, the most important thing to remember is that you can't meditate incorrectly because it is a practice. You're not supposed to clear all of your thoughts out of your mind because well, that's impossible. The point of meditation isn't to be thought-free. The point of meditation is to cultivate more presence with yourself.

I recommend meditating first thing in the morning so that it doesn't get away from you as the day progresses and also because it helps to set you up for dealing with any stressors that may arise during the day. You will be more connected to yourself and more equipped for not holding onto stress.

The intention with sitting meditation is to expand your capacity to hold space for yourself so your everyday life can become a living meditation practice.

MEDITATION RITUAL

Find a comfortable and quiet place to sit. Set a timer (I recommend the "Insight Timer" app) for twenty minutes and close your eyes. Take three deep breaths and feel your body and become aware of your senses. Notice any sensations in your body, any scents, any sounds. Then gently bring your attention to your breath or focus on the repetition of a one-word mantra such as Om, peace, or relax. *Every time you notice yourself thinking thoughts, bring your-self back to your breath or to your mantra, not as a way to stop thinking but as a way to practice observing your state of mind and being, and then making a choice to come back to yourself by making an adjustment to come back to your breath or mantra, all while practicing being compassionate and non-judgmental.*

If you visualize this process, it's a circular motion with the inhale and exhale and also the process of noticing the thoughts in your mind and gently, but firmly bringing yourself back to yourself. It's yin yang flow.

When the bell rings, take a moment to give thanks to Source energy and all of your loved ones that support you from the other side.

BEING A CONSCIOUS PRACTITIONER

In essence, being a conscious practitioner is living a life in a meditative state of creating and holding space for yourself. This doesn't mean you're walking around like a monk or a nun. It means that you are highly attuned and aware, and have the ability to make conscious choices throughout your day. It means that you are meeting yourself exactly where you are.

It's a place where you will go into an explorative medita-tive state. It's an adventure. A journey into unknown territory where you get to discover more about you and feel more of what's been living inside of you. It is not a linear process. It is a meditative process, therefore, fluid and intuitive. And you can't do it wrong because it's a practice. When you see life in this way, you will naturally see how you can impact your life by putting attention on moments that were either tossed aside or turned into something dramatic. Now don't get me wrong, it's not always easy or pretty. It's a practice! I love the word practice because it automatically implies that absolutely nothing has to be perfect. You are off the hook even before you even start. How amazing is that? We can just play!

I have broken down this conscious practitioner practice into six simple yet potent steps that can be used when an emotional, mental, or physical entry point is activated. Below is the general process but in follow three chapters, I share specific rituals for each realm.

At the core of this practice, you are cultivating a deeper level of compassion and love for yourself and others. Love is the energetic binding force.

1. CREATING SPACE

Declutter your life and practice being with yourself without distractions. Allowing yourself to feel whatever is present for you without reaching for your favorite way to disconnect from the moment. When you are filling your time with over-working, over-socializing, social media, TV, shopping, mental obsessions, over-focusing on other people, future-tripping, and engaging in mindless busy-work, a disconnect takes place because you are not allowing you to be with yourself. You are practicing avoidance. By not giving yourself moments of quiet and stillness, you make it extra challenging to digest and integrate all the things that are happening in your life. Then, all of those life experiences pile up in your system and you end up feeling stuffed and cranky. Many people have created a habit of being so busy and distracted that they don't even know how to slow down and create space for themselves. It's similar to having a habit of overeating to the point of feeling stuffed and not knowing how it feels to be satisfied because over-eating has been such an ingrained habit. If you haven't experienced something, how would you know what's possible on the other side?

Even though one of my clients had taken a bunch of self-development courses, she didn't really understand what it meant to create space for herself until we did a session together where I guided her through a series of breathing and visualization meditations. Up until that point she had been avoiding anything meditative because of her fear of the unknown. A fear of going into the depths of despair and not being able to come out of it, and then having to put on a happy face out in the world so she could be productive. The ironic part is that the avoidance of being present with herself was the real cause of her ongoing feelings of despair throughout her life. She had an 'aha' moment that she was confusing creating space with self-care activities. The self-care activities were still "doing" and not necessarily "being". It was another thing to check off the list, which is something she was great at.

In the process of guiding her to be present with herself, she had all these feelings of being out of control. Sweaty palms, racing heart, and anxiety went up. This is why she avoided meditation like the plague. Her inner child was fearful to be in this world again. It was safer to keep that tender part of her as well as her emotions hidden. And since her adult identity had been so wrapped up in her ability to be in control, her success and productivity were the perfect validation to continue along those lines. They were the perfect excuses *not* to create space.

Here's some suggestions of how to create time and space for yourself:

- Stop checking your phone and social media randomly. Use the "screen time" app on your phone to schedule allotted time for social media, etc. The average amount people check their phone is 80 times a day. Average amount of time on social media is 30 minutes a day which equals 22 days out of the year!
- Stop consuming information and start practicing what you already know.
- Slow down. Literally. With your movement, with your speech, with everything.
- Declutter your schedule and your to-do list of things that are not priorities.
- Take moments of deep breaths throughout the day at work.
- Take a walk without your phone.
- Walk slower and take in the environment around you.
- Dance breaks.
- Hire a nanny for a few hours during the week.

- Create a morning ritual of meditation and journaling to prepare you for your day.
- Create an evening ritual and shut down screens early to prepare your mind and body for sleep.
- Do one thing at a time (no multi-tasking).
- Say 'no' to anything you don't desire to do.
- Replace social media or TV time with you time.

A great resource on how to declutter your life and live a more quality existence is *Essentialism: The Disciplined Pursuit of Less* by Greg McKeown.

BEING WITH THE BREATH

Breath is the most simple and profound way to create space. The act of inhaling expands your chest and automatically creates space and exhaling grounds you. Conscious breathing brings both presence and concentration to the moment. There are many different types of breathing practices. Slow long breaths. Fast quick breaths. Hold the breath after inhaling. Counting your inhale and exhale count. To keep things simple here, I recommend you do a seven second count for each inhale and exhale when you're focusing on creating space with your breath, specifically.

A natural result of creating time and space is that you will have more awareness of your energy tank. Energy is our hottest commodity and it's important to treat it as such. In order to do this deep work, you need to pay special attention to your energy level. Most people are spending their energy endlessly when they are already on fumes, or close to it. Keep your tank full, and then you will have the energy you need to do this work and to live your fullest life.

You get to choose what you spend your energy on and how you fill your tank. Plus, the process in this book will organically support you in this. I used to waste my energy on resentment. That was my thing; you "did me wrong" (whether it was real or not). I would obsess about it and become resentful. No wonder I was tired all the time.

2. NOTICING

My dad shared the practice of noticing with me many years ago. He described it as imagining your physical self where it is in this moment and then your higher self is sitting on the top of a mountain looking down at physical yourself. This higher self sees everything with loving, clear eyes. She just watches and knows and trusts what is. She observes your thoughts, emotions, and behaviors.

It's a practice of mindfulness - paying attention to things that are changing. Life is constantly changing and there's always movement happening within you. The noticing of the changes is the actual work here, and you will find that your awareness and insights will increase. You'll notice more of your thoughts and feel more emotions and sensations. Noticing is an internal check-in and connecting to what's happening within you moment to moment. This will give you the ability to identify if an entry point has been activated, and when you're able to identify an entry point activation, you have the power to choose how to respond. You bring conscious choice to the moment versus being reactionary. With practice over time, your ability to notice the subtleties within you will increase.

NOTICING RITUAL

As you are doing your normal day-to-day activities, notice how you are feeling, ask yourself what you are thinking, and check in to see how your body is feeling. Continue to do this check-in throughout the day. You don't need to address anything or change anything that is happening. Just observe yourself.

After each check-in, thank yourself for taking a moment to be with yourself in this new way.

3. ATTENTION

Have you noticed that what you focus your attention on seems to become magically more meaningful or even larger? Our attention is our biggest asset because we have *complete* control over it. We can choose what we focus on. That's completely our choice. No one can climb into your mind and tell you what to think. This can be good or bad depending on your perspective.

It's good when you realize that you have power over your life. It's bad when you'd rather be in victim consciousness. For example, if you notice that you're obsessing about whether this one person likes you or not, you can turn your attention toward all the loving friendships you have in your life. It's better than if you choose to stalk their social media to try to find "evidence" that they hate you.

There's no way that you will ever be able to control what other people think, feel, or do. But you do have control over what you think, feel, and do. And that's a gift. When you achieve this clarity, you then have the power to change your life.

As a race, we excel at being distracted. Our culture of multi-tasking, rushing, and technological over-stimulation has made this even more of a reality. Have you noticed that your thoughts jump all over and you have absolutely no control over your mind? This is a result of practicing being distracted for your entire life. The good news is that just as you have created a habit of distraction, you can create a new habit of focusing your attention. It's like building a new muscle. You can't expect that going to the gym every now and then is going to build the muscles you want. It's going to take consistency and practice. Not just in sitting meditation but in life – 24/7. That might sound daunting, but the alternative is being dependent on your uncontrollable mind, and you know how that feels – not so good. Imagine what's possible when you have control over what you put your attention on. The possibilities are endless.

The way you cultivate your attention is through sitting meditation and by putting your undivided attention on one thing. When you notice yourself being distracted, you bring your attention back to the subject. This means that you are practicing extending the amount of time you keep your awareness on something or someone. This requires you to do one thing at a time, which brings us back to creating space. It could be with your thoughts, in a conversation, with a project, at work, in any situation. And since you're able to witness what's happening within you, you can see what you want to put your attention on.

Some examples of how to cultivate your attention:

- Looking at anything for an extended period of time, such as, watching the faucet drip.
- Repeat the same mantra over and over.
- Focusing on how your breath feels going in and out of your nose.
- If you're obsessing, put your attention on another thought.

Keep practicing, no matter what, because in order for you to release your physical and emotional weight, you will have to surrender to the fact that the only thing you can control is you and nothing else. Which means that it's in your best interest to cultivate your ability to concentrate your mind, otherwise it will run amok.

4. CURIOSITY

Having a childlike, beginner's mind will serve you in this practice and in life. Being able to be in a place of inquiry and exploration completely shifts the vibration of the adventure. Imagine being in a new country which you have never stepped foot in before. What happens when you enter with an air of wonder and fascination versus when you enter with closed mindedness and indifference? There's an openness to the unknown, which means there's less gripping on to an predicted outcome. You start to see things in an entirely different way than you were able to before. For example, you realize that what you've been so adamant about believing, isn't actually true. You discover that you have created an entire life based on a false belief. You uncover answers that you never knew you even had questions for. You come across emotions that were hidden in the crevices and now you can hold them. You actively engage with your body instead of ignoring it because you truly want to unearth what's lying beneath the surface. There's a receptivity to new possibilities. Your willingness increases. When you are in a state of inquiry, the entire Universe opens up to you and delivers answers that may surprise you. Your intuitive 'spidey senses' grow because now there's spaciousness to expand into. When you are curious, it means that you are willing to see, hear, or feel something different than what you've ever seen, heard, or felt before.

When you lack curiosity, it's like you're living in a box and completely shut down with tunnel vision. It's telling the Universe that you are not open to expanding because the box you're in is exactly what you want.

Intelligent women have a challenging time releasing what they know, or what they think they know, because that intelligence has created their successes and life as they know it. It was humbling when I realized that I was blocking myself with my emotional and spiritual intelligence. Curiosity is the antidote to this because it shows that you are receptive to learning and when you are truly open to learning, teachers, answers, and help always comes. You will serendipitously see a book that you haven't paid attention to in years and find that it's exactly what you needed to read in that moment. Or you will hear someone say something that rings true and answers a question that you've been pondering for days.

INNER CHILD RITUAL

Do you remember when you were young and curious? This is the energy that I'm talking about. Your inner child wants to explore. Let her. Take some time to reflect on a moment when you were young and playful, where you were curious about something you'd never experienced before. Imagine yourself in that space. Were you home or in the park or in school? What did your hair look like? What were you wearing? Who was around? Now put yourself into that little child's body and see through her eyes. Feel the sense of exploration, excitement, and anticipation she might be feeling. Connect with her right now. Connect with her sense of curiosity. Notice how she is experiencing life as an adventure. Notice her openness and willingness to play.

Once you feel complete, thank your inner child for showing you what's possible when we open up to curiosity. Thank yourself, your higher power, and your loved ones on the other side for holding space for you to connect with the little one in you.

5. PIVOTING

I love something else my dad taught me years ago. He explained that when you make a one-degree shift, you end up on a completely different trajectory. Just one-degree has that big of an impact. And just like all meditations, the power lies in the *subtleties*. This is not about making big moves or forcing yourself to be where you are not. It's about tuning into the nuance of where you are in the moment and making a conscious choice to lean into the juiciest spot that will reconnect you to yourself, not an outcome.

When you notice yourself veering off the flow, you can make an adjustment. Adjustments are such a powerful act of awareness and choice, and it's usually the sum of the small adjustments that you make over time that will end up making the biggest impact. For most people, it's challenging to make a big adjustment unless they have already done the work to make a big turn. But it is realistic to be able to make a bunch of small turns. As you practice, you will build your muscle and in time you will be able to make bigger and bigger adjustments. The key is to meet yourself wherever you are.

Imagine you're driving a car down a two-lane street and you want to make U-turn. You're going to have to slow down and make small adjustments in order to turn the car around. The same is true for your state of mind and being.

If you're feeling anxious and overwhelmed, you can ask yourself, what tweak can I make right now that will put me in a spot that feels more in alignment? In the past your adjustment might have been to tell yourself to calm down. That is a good example of how making too big of a pivot can put you even more out of alignment because you are bypassing what is being asked of you in that moment. Perhaps the perfect pivot would be to take five deep breaths. Perhaps the perfect pivot would be crying your eyes out. Perhaps the perfect pivot would be to take at big leap of faith. The pivot step forces you to really tune in with where you are and what you are needing. What's that sweet spot? That sweet spot might be to make a sharp turn. It all depends on where you are and the only way you'll know is by practicing this meditative process and learning about yourself as you go.

I had a client who was always trying to do everything "right" and always trying to "figure things out". She was trying too hard. So, I told her straight up, "You're doing too much!" I then told her about the pivoting tool. It was the thing that shifted everything for her because she was able to see how she was trying to make these huge turns when all she needed to do was just make a tiny one or two-degree shift. Many times, that shift was simply putting her attention on her breath in the moment. She was amazed at how much this tiny pivot decreased her anxiety and increased her calmness, clarity, and well-being.

PIVOTING RITUAL

The most important aspect in choosing a pivot honors where you are in a particular moment. The perfect thing that will bring you back closer to your body and presence. It could literally be anything. But here's a list of powerful pivots in moments where you are really struggling:

- *Breath.*
- *Dance break.*
- *Talk a walk and feel your feet with every step and take in the nature around you.*
- *Choose another thought that is closer to alignment that is believable to you in that moment.*
- *Put your hands on your heart and tell yourself, "It's ok to feel this emotion right now."*

When you choose to pivot in a resonant way, you will find yourself closer to alignment. This gives you the ability to make another conscious choice to pivot after that and so on. You are making one tweak after another and as you practice you will find that you are able to make larger and larger pivots over time.

6. DIGESTION

What I know to be true is that humans need time to digest their experiences in order to integrate and metabolize what they have learned. Imagine being at a buffet, and you are stuffing yourself silly with delicious food. You are full but you keep putting food in your mouth. What happens? You feel sick, and now the potentially amazing experience has become a disaster because when you overstuff yourself, even when it's absolutely delicious, you're going to get overly full. But why wait until you're overly full? Take the time to digest so you can really take in each experience as it comes. And being aware of your capacity is not only going to help you in your real-life eating journey but also in your internal processes. If you are in the practice of noticing, you will be able to identify how full you are, emotionally and physically.

If you think about the actual digestive system, it needs time to rest and digest. That fasting period in between each meal allows your body to recover and integrate all the nutrients into your system. It takes energy for your body to break down the food you eat and transport the good stuff and the waste to where they need to go. If you keep eating every two hours, you will overwork your system. Your body will be confused about if it's ok to relax because it's clocking in overtime. The exact same process is true for your emotional body. So much happens in one day. Think about that. You need to digest all the occurrences, feelings, and events in your life every single day. Especially if you're a woman who is committed to growth, you are going to experience multiple transitions. Transitions are the places where most people get stuck because they're entering into a new experience and that can increase anxiety and the ability to trust themselves as well as the process. This is where digestion comes in to assist you because just as when you feel physically stuffed you experience unpleasant symptoms, the same can be true for our experiences. When you don't digest your life you can become what I like to call energetically constipated! Digestion can happen in many different ways. Personally, my favorites are: gratitude, celebration, and seeing the good in the "bad". These tools will keep you flowing. They are like energetic probiotics!

GRATITUDE RITUAL

Start a gratitude practice by writing what you're grateful for in your journal every day. Write three every morning and every night. But don't stop there. As you move through the world, you will come across endless things to be grateful for. Take a moment to say "thank you" when something happens that lights up your gratitude juices. The key is to feel the gratitude in your body and to let it expand until you can feel it throughout your entire being. This is the secret sauce. It's not enough to just write it, say it or think it. You must feel it.

Examples of gratitude:

- *I am grateful for the stranger that held the door for me.*
- *I am grateful that I found the perfect parking spot.*
- *I am grateful that I am feeling good in my body.*
- *I am grateful I took the time to take a bath today instead of my to-do's.*
- *I am grateful that I said "I love you" to my partner today even when I was upset.*
- *I am grateful for the sun shining on my face.*
- *I am grateful for a warm, safe home.*

The second way I love to digest is by celebrating. I suggest celebrating everything and by everything, I mean all the big and the small wins. Nothing is too small to celebrate, nothing! Milestones don't have to be something big like running a marathon. Celebration simply means that you did something that you've never done before and if that means you were able to meditate for the first time, you ran for one minute, you chose not to emotionally eat when you normally would have, or you stopped and connected with yourself before reacting, those are all moments to celebrate and celebrate hard.

When I first started a celebration practice, every time I notice a "negative" thought, I would celebrate. This is radical in so many ways because we are conditioned to beat ourselves up when we see that we're doing something "bad" or not nice to ourselves or others. But I celebrated because I was so excited that I could see things that I didn't see before. That's huge. I kept reminding myself that this is a process, and a process means that every step, moment, and choice I make makes a difference.

I recall a moment when I ran my first and only a 5k race. It was freezing cold by the water, and I didn't hit my goal time of ten minutes a mile. These thoughts came up telling me that I didn't train hard enough and that I failed. But then I caught myself in that moment and decided to celebrate me completing the race in inclement weather and for noticing my judgement while it was happening. The ability to celebrate my judgements opened up a space to get to know myself better. These micro-moments are more powerful than you realize because they add up and create momentum.

CELEBRATION RITUAL

Celebrate by journaling about all the accomplishments you've made, share your wins with your friends and community, have a fun celebratory dance break, or look in the mirror and connect with your eyes and say with love, "I am so proud of you", just as you would to your best friend, partner, or family member. And again, feel it. Get giddy! Because you just did something that you've never done before or thought you would never be able to do. And that's big. Yay you. Applaud yourself. Make up a cheer with your name in it.

Examples of celebrating wins:

- *I celebrate that I started dating again!*
- *I celebrate that I noticed a new limiting belief!*
- *I celebrate that I listened to my intuition and it was spot on!*
- *I celebrate creating a boundary at work!*
- *I celebrate that I didn't feel compelled to eat the donuts at work while I was stressed out!*
- *I celebrate that I meditate daily now!*
- *I celebrate saying thank you when someone complimented me!*
- *I celebrate sharing more of myself with my friends!*

While writing this book, I would celebrate after I finished writing each chapter or when I managed to get through a section that felt extra challenging to write. I would typically jump on my trampoline while yelling out to my mirror, "You did it!! Yayy! I'm so proud of you!". Other times I would take a dance break to whatever song I was in the mood for. And sometimes I would simply feel the joy inside of me and really allow myself fully marinate in the yumminess of my accomplishment.

Become a miner of the good when "bad" things happen by training yourself to look for good in places you normally wouldn't look. For example, I was completely devastated when a more recent boyfriend broke up with me a few months ago out of nowhere. I let myself feel my feelings and grieve the relationship. I did the mental work of questioning the limiting thoughts that were arising in me, and I made sure to take extra care of myself physically. But I also chose to see the bird's-eye view, that his letting me go was the thing that propelled me into the next level of my purpose work and is why I'm writing this very book. I grieved him and mined the experience for gold simultaneously! The more you are able to do this with big heartbreaks or tiny slights and annoyances the more tapped in you are, and when you're tapped in, everything that happens in your life can be digested and you can take in whatever nourishment is available.

Being a conscious practitioner is a moment-based practice, not an outcome-based practice. This isn't about making something happen in the ways that we expect them to. It's about feeling, listening, and then acting on those internal intuitive instincts. We all have them – we just need to listen. A lot of times the reason why people have a hard time listening is that the ego can be so loud that it becomes like a radio station playing all the time in your head. But you don't realize it because it's been on all your life. This process will help you have control over that radio dial.

CHAPTER 6

GO THROUGH, NOT AROUND

(THE EMOTIONAL REALM)

*"I imagine one of the reasons people cling to their hates
so stubbornly is because they sense, once hate is gone, they will be
forced to deal with pain."*
— James Baldwin

Even though I was a super aware and an emotionally intelligent woman that did a ton of personal work, there was more to be revealed. I know many women who think that they are in touch with their emotions but are still lacking an intimate, transparent, and vulnerable relationship with themselves. This may seem hard to imagine, but our minds are very tricky and will do anything to keep us from being with ourselves.

The path of alchemy is a path of holding yourself to the highest level of compassion and approval. There is no freedom in forcing, pressuring, worrying, controlling, or expecting yourself to do anything. That is the old you. You are entering into a new space of discovering the real you by shedding layers of backed up emotions from years of repression. This is the you that has been here all along but has been waiting for you to own it. It's a new paradigm of trusting yourself: Radical trust.

When we are connected to our emotions, we are able to connect deeper with our intuition. Emotions are not bad, they are entry points, and when they are activated, they tell us exactly where we are and what we need, much like a compass. Once you build a new relationship with your emotions, you will learn to trust their guidance. I thought I was doing the emotional work, because I was emotional. Just because you're emotional doesn't mean you're doing the emotional work. Those are two different things. And so what I noticed in my process was that I was a child emotionally, and I was in victimhood state of mind a great deal of the time. I was letting the little girl in me, who was hurt and angry, lead instead of a mature, grounded adult.

Signs that you are emotionally immature:

- You don't hold yourself accountable for your actions and blame others.
- You're fearful about everything and expect things to shift without doing the work.
- You try to control and manipulate the people or experiences around you so you can get your preferred outcome.
- You are unable to see your projections onto others.

- You are resentful all the time because you are expecting others to change to fit your needs.
- You use your *woe is me* stories to get attention from others by way of colluding and commiserating.
- You self-sabotage almost anything that has the potential for joy and fulfillment.

Signs that you're emotionally mature:

- You are accountable for your actions and look deep within yourself.
- You trust the process and are willing to do the work.
- You allow people to be who they are and are able to accept them along with all of the experiences in your life.
- You see how you project onto others and use that clarity to see deeper parts of yourself.
- You are a sovereign being because you know that you have no control over other people. You are able to keep the focus on you.
- You are attracted to people who will tell you the truth when you are off balance.
- You are aware when the ego wants to self-sabotage and you use the necessary tools to make sure you don't allow it to.
- You're learning how to become an adult that holds space for your inner child so that you can more masterfully hold space for yourself in the grittiest of moments when the immature parts of you want to act out or hide.

PAIN VERSUS SUFFERING

Pain is different than suffering. Pain is part of feeling. Pain is inevitable. The experience of pain is what comes with being a human being. It's part of our experience. Things are going to happen in our lives that we cannot control and we will feel pain. Suffering however, is an entirely different animal.

Suffering is when we believe the stories, conditioning, thoughts, and beliefs that are created by our ego that keep us spinning. Suffering keeps us from feeling the deeper emotions. But the good news is that you can choose *not* to suffer even though the pain is there. You can do this instead:

- Identify whether you are in pain or in suffering.
- If you are in pain, feel your emotions (emotional realm).
- If you are suffering, question your thoughts and limiting beliefs (mental realm, next chapter).

Recently, in addition to my devastating and sudden breakup, two of my sweet furry family members, my dog, Ceba, and cat, Baby, recently passed. Each time, I noticed how my ego was creating a story that I could have done things differently in their last days, weeks, or months, telling me I should have done this or that. The guilt was unbearable. Now, that is suffering. I noticed that I was going down this road of self-inflicted suffering, so I started to question the thoughts that my ego was trying to feed me as truth. From this questioning, it became clear that I was creating this feeling of guilt because I was avoiding feeling the raw emotions underneath, the grief. That is pain.

The ego creates lies (suffering) in order to protect you from feeling the emotions (pain). Visually, I see the energy of the raw emotions hiding in the darkest, smallest spaces in my gut and the lies are like a damp blanket covering them in order to keep you from entering those hidden spaces.

After I was able to see the truth of what was happening, I had another moment of clarity. In choosing to suffer, I was keeping myself disconnected from myself and disconnected from Ceba and Baby's spirits. When I was able to see that, I opened myself up to feel all of my grief. In the midst of feeling that pain was a sense of pleasure, pleasure in the renewed connection to myself and to my furry family on the other side. By the end, I was able to see the truth of the entire experience – that I did my very best and created a loving space for them to pass humanely and in peace.

So, I want you to check in with yourself and ask if you are connecting with your emotions or are you creating suffering? Use your emotions as the powerful entry point that they are. Trust your emotions. They are going to guide you to exactly where you need to be to reveal who you really are.

When you have this awareness about the difference between pain and suffering, it's like swimming in the ocean with goggles. You finally have the necessary equipment. You can move through your day inquiring where you are on the spectrum and can see if you're trying to control your emotions or if you are letting them move through you. So it's really important to understand the distinction between the two because then you will be able to identify where you are, which gives you the power to choose how you will respond. If you don't have this clarity, you are moving through your experiences blindly.

People think that feeling emotions means that you're out of flow. I disagree! When you're tuned into yourself and able to be present with what's wanting to be felt in that moment, you're actually in flow. And once you allow yourself to feel what needs to be felt, the emotions just blow through like the wind. And then that wind will come back again at another time and you let it blow through again. But if you're resisting it, you will feel the wrath of suffering consistently.

DEALING WITH PAIN

No one wants to feel pain, but the irony is that we must feel pain in order to expand and grow. If we don't feel our underlying pain, we get stuck in the exact spot where the pain occurred in the first place, until we feel and release it. That's why there are so many adults who act like children. They got stuck there because no one taught them how to process their emotions. That repressed pain ends up being expressed, or acted out, in their current lives.

I know this story all too well. I would rage on my exes when our relationship reached a deeper level of intimacy and commitment. I never raged on anyone else but them because my younger self, who was raped, would act out of fear whenever someone got too close. The shame and fear were still in my system. Rage protects the shameful spots and I didn't know how to deal with any of it.

It's better to feel it now rather than later because pain always finds a way out. When we feel it as close to real-time as possible, it's actually easier to process because there will be less build-up of emotional layers that have been accumulated, numbed, accumulated, numbed, and so on. It's similar to plaque build-up. When you don't floss daily, you will get layers of plaque that will require more work to get rid of it, and if you wait too long, the dental hygienist may have to bring out the big guns. When you allow yourself to feel and move through the pain, as it arises, you are giving yourself a gift. You are honoring yourself in such a powerful way. You are saying to yourself, "I love you and I trust that you can handle this". And as a result, you will then have the space to do the mental work. But if you are constipated with pain, there's no room to ingest anything else, even the good stuff in your life.

Trauma has a way of being stored in your body, especially when you go through the aftermath alone. I didn't realize I was experiencing trauma when I was young, so I didn't have the language or the understanding to express what was happening to me or inside of me. I just knew I wanted to disappear. For years, I used food, alcohol, weed, relationships, and most of all, my addiction to suffering and drama to shield me from all of my underlying feelings.

I didn't know how to process my emotions, because I was not taught how to process my emotions. That's not something they teach in school. It's not something that a lot of parents know how to do. So it's okay that we have repressed emotions and these layers that have been built up. But now that we're adults, we can choose to feel those things now. And so it's going to take you creating space to hold yourself at a new level of compassion and stillness. Stillness needs to be there in order to feel, especially if you're constantly busy in your life and in your mind.

I had this interesting mix of being emotionally intelligent, because of my empathy, but also being incredibly emotionally immature and out of control because of my inability to connect with the parts of me that needed love and care. It wasn't until I stopped using my numbing agents that I was able to truly feel, and to be vulnerable and transparent with myself.

Some common numbing agents are food, social media, work, relationships, or the obsession with or over-use of anything like alcohol, drugs, or exercise – basically, anything that you are using to distract yourself from feeling. But the one that slides under the radar the most is the addiction to suffering and drama. It is highly effective at numbing because most people have a hard time seeing that they are attached to suffering. I invite you to identify your numbing agents and start to release them in your own time. Then observe what emotions arise from this work because they most definitely will. That's why the numbing agent is there in the first place – to keep you from feeling.

Releasing your shame is like freeing your imprisoned inner child. Take that in for a moment. Can you see her? She has been locked up in a cage for who knows how long and now you courageously have gone into the dark dungeon-like space, put the key in the lock, and set her free. At first, she will be terrified and at a complete loss for how to feel or exist in the world outside of this cage. But as you hold her and love her, she will start to relax and heal. That's how it felt for me when I realized I was ignoring my inner child. When I reconnected with her, I was able to nourish her in the ways she desperately needed for decades. We built a new relationship solidified in trust and connection. And since time isn't linear, when your inner child feels safe and loved, so do you.

Shame is an epidemic in our country and in the world at large. As a collective, we do not want to go close to it, wouldn't touch it with a ten-foot pole, as if it's contagious. We act as though if we allow ourselves to connect with shame, then maybe other people will see it in us, and that makes us too vulnerable. Or they will avoid us because they're afraid that they'll get stuck in the darkness, but the truth is that you remain stuck in a limbo state of suffering if you don't go there.

In order to heal shame, you must travel into the deepest parts of you that lack compassion, the parts that are pitch dark, and introduce forgiveness because shame cannot survive where compassion lives.

BEING WITH YOUR EMOTIONS RITUAL

- *It all begins with noticing when an emotional entry point is activated – an emotion starts to bubble up. You feel some sadness arising - or loneliness, or irritation. When you identify that this is happening, create space with a clear and loving intention of healing.*

- *Go to a quiet place that feels safe, even if that's the bathroom stall at work. Be courageous by giving yourself permission to feel what's coming up for you and surrender to the experience. Be kind to yourself if fears arise or loud voices enter your mind. It's as if you are holding a baby in your arms – it's that sacred of an experience, even if it's for five minutes on the Q train. You are that sacred. When we create this type of space, it already starts the process of healing because loving attention is being put on healing.*

- *Whether you're standing or sitting, begin by closing your eyes and get in your body by taking three deep breaths into your lower abdomen and feel the breath move through you. Then be still and be in the silence and presence of the moment and feel what is arising in you.*

- *Are emotions bubbling up? Are childhood memories entering into your visions? Do you hear words popping in? Whatever is coming up, put your soft attention onto it with an energy of curiosity.*

- *Allow whatever it is to guide you to the next thing that wants to arise. Perhaps it's another emotion or another memory. It's as if you're on a ride. Don't force it. Surrender to it. Be with it. You may feel an urge to distract yourself, but just gently bring yourself back to the emotions that are wanting attention.*

- *Tears may fall or not. Be compassionate with yourself however you react to what arises. Hold space for yourself as if you were holding space for your dearest friend or family member.*

- *Once you feel complete, put both of your hands on your heart and put your attention on your heart space. Thank your heart for being so open and so brave during this experience and express whatever else wants to be shared with your heart. And tell your heart that you will come back to this space whenever your heart needs you.*

- *Then take three deeps breaths to reconnect with your body. Take a moment to thank the Universe, your ancestors, and loved ones on the other side for all of their love, holding, and guidance. And then slowly open your eyes.*

- *Journal about your experience so you can digest what just happened. Insights, images, words, feelings, memories. Write freely without too much thought. Let your hands do the writing. Then take your time transitioning into what you need to do next.*

You'll know that you are creating a more intimate relationship with your heart space when you will feel more comfortable being with yourself without a need for distraction when you're in discomfort. You will feel more comfortable feeling your emotions and will start to crave presence and self-forgiveness. You will be able to hold yourself with exquisite attention and love and notice more easily when you're not. You will be able to be radically honest with yourself about things that you have been hiding. You will start to slow down and learn what your personal pace is and honor it. You will not expect others to take care of you but will receive their love graciously when it is offered.

FORGIVENESS

Many times we can feel our emotions but we still haven't forgiven. Women who are hiding behind their weight, and people in general, are not that forgiving. They're holding on to so much resentment. And that's part of the weight that you're going to release in order to release your body armor.

As long as I can remember, I would hold grudges toward other people. There was so much resentment in me. But the day that I realized that all of that resentment was really directed at myself is when I really started to forgive. I finally felt the pain that I had caused myself throughout my life. I saw how my lack of self-forgiveness was not only hurting me but my relationships because the way we feel toward ourselves is projected onto the outside world in some shape or form. It's a direct correlation – no exceptions. Everyone is my mirror and an entry point into my power.

In my acupuncture practice, I wasn't only supporting my patients in their journeys – they also supported my growth by reflecting onto me exactly what I needed to see in myself. About six years ago, I had a patient that would come in every week feeling overwhelmed with her spinning mind. I felt stressed when I saw her because I wasn't making the impact that I hoped for. No suggestions I offered ever helped her, and I felt inadequate. I questioned myself and my ability to hold space for another person's growth. But then there was a moment when I saw that I was internally projecting my ideas of "success" onto her by being disappointed in her process. I saw how this was about me and my own feelings of not being enough and trying to get a sense of worthiness by helping others. She unknowingly reflected my own spinning mind and inability to be present with what was happening at that time. It was humbling and empowering to see my reflection and my projections. That experience shifted my entire acupuncture practice and how I hold space for my patients. I'm able to notice in a split second if my ego is wanting to make it about me or if I'm really holding space for them with unwavering love.

If we stay open to seeing things differently, a whole new world opens for us. We start to see that the things we've been saying or thinking about others are what we are thinking about ourselves. It takes an open mind and a shift in perspective to be able to see this, but if we start paying attention to what we are thinking about others, we have a huge opportunity to go deeper into our power.

Forgiveness starts by being able to take responsibility and not put our stuff onto others. We see the clear delineation in our boundaries. That's your garden, this is my garden, and I'm going to stay over here, tend to my veggies, and leave yours alone.

Once we are able to see our boundaries clearly, we can redirect our attention, that was directed outward, back toward us, not with blame or judgment but with clarity and love. We choose to see with radical honesty how we have either hurt others or hurt ourselves. We make a choice to release all the ways that we have been unkind. We make a list of the people

we've hurt, including ourselves, and we own up to what we did
that was unkind, and direct loving energy toward them/us.

FORGIVENESS RITUAL

- *Make a list of all the people you are resentful toward or are not
  on good terms with.*
- *One at a time, write down why you are resentful toward each
  one of them.*
- *Write down what part you played in each circumstance. Your
  thoughts or behaviors that added to the disconnection.*
- *Write down what you could have done instead.*
- *Take a moment to ask yourself if you are willing to forgive them.*
- *Take a moment to ask yourself if you are willing to forgive
  yourself.*
- *Sit with the emotions arising and see if you can feel some love
  bubbling up in you.*
- *Burn the paper and say out loud, "I forgive you" and "I for-
  give myself".*
- *When you feel complete, thank yourself for being so courageous
  in this act of releasing blame.*

Whenever there's shame, anger, or guilt, forgiveness is a
potent medicine. You may not notice it now if you tend to
numb or distract yourself from feeling pain, but there's usually
blame and resentment lurking around it. When we are able to
be present with the pain, space is created for the blame to arise.
When you see the blame, it is usually toward the other person

because it's easier for us to blame others. Look at what you are blaming other people for and use that as an entry point into seeing your reflection in that mirror. Most of the time I see that I am actually resentful toward myself, but I displaced the resentment onto them. That's why I focus on self-forgiveness because when we are able to do this, we will naturally be able to forgive others as a result of this internal work. It's more effective to go straight to the root when pulling out a weed versus having to cut the branches over and over.

I find that self-forgiveness is the most powerful way to develop an intimate relationship with yourself. When you emotionally eat, are you judging yourself or are you being compassionate with yourself? Forgiveness is required for all situations where you are being unkind to yourself, from emotionally eating after a stressful day to yelling at someone and feeling guilty about it after.

Guilt is a state of mind, not an emotion. It's your ego telling you that you did something wrong. It's a series of thoughts that are leading you down a road of rumination and suffering. The interesting part is that your ego can tell you that you did something wrong for absolutely anything, even for things that are completely made up by your imagination. Someone doesn't call you back, you create a story that you must have done something wrong, and then you feel guilty. But really, they are just busy with a project. Then, when you add food into the mix or not exercising, you create a story that you are not doing it right because in your mind you think it's supposed to be done

one specific way, the "right" way. That's why guilt happens, because your perspective is skewed and tight like a narrow tunnel, where there's only one option and you are completely and utterly committed to it.

This was me. Guilt ran my world. I created stories upon stories that were not true. And as a result, I drove myself crazy with drama in my head along with countless hours of feeling guilty.

When we forgive ourselves, we are using that experience to get to know ourselves more. We consciously look at what's happening under the surface and question why we are feeling so bad about what happened.

When we forgive ourselves for big or small things, current or past experiences, it adds up and increases our capacity to love ourselves and others. When we are able to be kind and compassionate with ourselves in the spaces where we have previously gripped onto blame, we are able to extend that same compassion onto others, whether it's a stranger who cuts you off while driving or a loved one who did something deeply hurtful.

> *"Forgiveness is for yourself because it frees you. It lets you out of that prison you put yourself in."*
> — Louise Hay

EMBODIMENT

This is like the Ph.D. in honoring your emotions and being so right with how you feel that you own all of it by embodying it all. You may want to do more of the Being With Your Emotions Ritual above before practicing this or you may feel ready to go for it. Trust your instincts.

Embodiment happens when you are able to be in tune with your emotions and let them guide you to move your body in intuitive ways that express how you feel. It requires deep listening and connection with your emotions and your body.

The process is the same as the Being With Your Emotions Ritual except there are two extra steps. While you are in the midst of feeling whatever is arising in you, you may or may not feel an urge to move your body. If you're having a challenging time getting the juices flowing, you can put on music that will inspire you.

Free your mind and just let the emotions guide you to move or emote whatever wants to come out. You might feel like a weirdo. That means you're doing it right! Let go and surrender to your emotions. Express yourself in your facial expressions, your bodily movements, your voice. Imagine you're a child without the burden of cultural expectations. Claim your freedom and just go for it: Cry, wail, scream, curse, stomp around, punch the couch, do an interpretative dance. Whatever wants to come up and out is perfection. When you feel complete, before you do the closing hands on your heart portion of the ritual, move your hips in circles. Feel your juiciness and 'turn-on' throughout your body.

I want to share with you how I have used this ritual to help me continue to process my grief over the loss of my pets. As I was sitting in my living room writing the first draft of this book and started to feel flutters of sadness arise, it was subtle at first, but as I focused my attention on it, the sadness expanded. So, I sat with it. Then I heard a super subtle inner voice telling me to move my body. So, I got up and let my body do whatever it wanted to do. I danced, crouched down, moaned in agony, swung my arms up in the air as if I was asking for help from the Universe. I just kept listening to what my body needed, moment by moment. Then, out of nowhere, I stopped and stood there in the middle of my living room in stillness with my hands over my heart with tears pouring out of my eyes. None of this was particularly graceful or pretty, but it expressed exactly how I felt at that moment.

This exercise was a sacred act of love. I was honoring my grief, myself, and the journey of being human. When we ignore this part of us, and don't give it any expression, we are ignoring the depths of our humanity. But when we choose to embody the beauty that is our emotions, we are alchemizing our pain into love, which expands our ability to receive love and abundance in our lives. It expands the amount of love we can give. It expands the amount of gratitude we feel for the entire spectrum of life. Our cup can be filled.

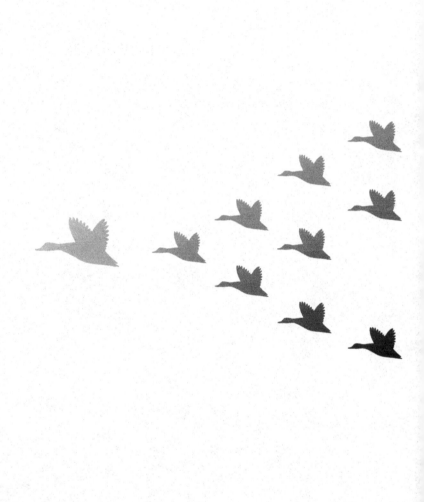

CHAPTER 7

REWIRING YOUR BRAIN

(THE MENTAL REALM)

"Don't believe everything you think."
— Byron Katie

It's a whole new world when we see with clear eyes. No veil. No matrix. No kidding. The ego is a tricky little thing and will do anything to convince you of its lies, brainwash your mind, and sabotage you. It convinces you that you are unworthy and unlovable, and you believe it as if it's the truth. Most people are living their lives based on worn out identities which no longer serve them. It's like they're living in 2020 with an old-school IBM computer. It's time to upgrade your hard drive!

Perhaps you have forgotten that your body is beautiful and perfect because there is only one of you. There is no one else in this world that has come close to being you, both inside and out! Not only that, there will never be anyone in the future that will even come close to being exactly like you. Do you understand that if you were willing to see things differently that everything in your life could, and would, change, including your physical body?

Your thoughts wire your brain into a specific pattern of thinking and ultimately determine how you feel and how you live your life. Over time, when you repeat the same negative thoughts to yourself about your body and appearance or about money, relationships, sex, or family you will eventually wire your brain to believe it as if it were written in stone. The good news is that you can also rewire your brain to believe new thoughts and beliefs. Your beliefs create your life. What lens or filter are you using? If you're not sure, you can actually find out by observing the reality of your mind right now. Be still and listen.

Do you have control over your mind or do you feel most comfortable in victim consciousness? It's so easy to get comfortable in a chaotic mind especially if it's your normal state of being. If you've never been taught how to concentrate and focus your mind, you probably haven't experienced what it feels like to have peace of mind. When you don't know what you're missing, you don't know what's possible.

ADDICTED TO SUFFERING

When I realized that I was addicted to suffering, it was like I woke up from a bad dream and entered into reality. It literally reminded me of the character Neo after taking the red pill and waking up in reality and out of the matrix. Actually seeing how I was creating drama in my life and in my mind as a way to not be present and live my fullest life was a rude awakening. At first it was humbling because I couldn't believe it took me so long to see it. How did I miss this when it was right in front of my face? Looking back it was glaringly obvious: I was creating drama left and right. I couldn't stop obsessing about what other people thought about me, about what was wrong with me, about what I did wrong... blah blah blah. But that's what happens when you're addicted to something. You can't see past that addiction. You just want that next hit. Those hits kept me from taking full responsibility over my mind and my life. Living that way kept me from being in my power. It kept me in hiding, and from radiating my light.

So when I saw this addiction; when I faced it and owned it, everything changed. I was able to notice when I was getting hooked by my temptress ego and *choose* to not go down that route because my pleasure, joy, and peace were more important than my outworn habitual need for suffering. The more I practiced this the easier it became, because I began to feel just how precious my peace of mind is and I was no longer willing to abandon it.

Once I emerged from my former self-inflicted matrix, I went cold turkey from my old M.O. and there were no withdrawal symptoms. Nope! Instead, I felt lighter and authentically in control of myself and my choices for the first time in my life. It was a miracle an utter game-changer.

Now I ask you, can you see how you are addicted to suffering and drama? Go ahead and take a closer look.

EGO TRAINING

One of the many jobs I've had throughout my life was as a dog trainer. What I learned was that it is most effective to give a command to stop a "negative" behavior while the dog is thinking about doing it. The second most effective is giving the command in the midst of the act, and the least effective is after the target behavior has already taken place.

In order to be an effective trainer you must be one step ahead of the dog. You must be aware at all times while potty training them. I remember when Ceba was a puppy and I could tell when she was about to try going potty by the way she started looking around, sniffing, and walking. The more I observed her, the more frequently I was able to catch her before she went potty inside.

After working this way with Ceba, everyone who met her mentioned how well trained she was. It's also important to be loving, calm, and assertive like Cesar Millan, the Dog Whisperer, says.

Now imagine your ego is the dog. As you practice training your ego, you must have a calm and assertive energy when it is acting out. Fighting or berating the ego for unwanted behaviors will probably backfire and it's not its fault anyway; the ego is just doing what it was created to do. And just how many people blame the dog when they have unwanted behaviors? People do the same thing with their egos. In reality, it's actually the human's responsibility to be the loving, calm, and assertive alpha. The ego is just doing what it does. You are the one who is responsible to be one step ahead of it, watching it.

I love this quote from Cesar because it illustrates the nature of the ego, *"If you give only eighty percent leadership, your dog will give you eighty percent following. And the other twenty percent of the time he will run the show. If you give your dog any opportunity for him to lead you, he will take it."*

As you practice, eventually you too will be able to be a step ahead of your ego and you will be able to avoid sabotaging behaviors altogether. With practice, you will learn how draw firm and loving boundaries with yourself.

MARTYR STORY AND BOUNDARIES

Everything is a mirror. Everything, whether it's a person or situation, is an opportunity to see ourselves. Everything shows us a reflection of who we are, or what we're going through, or what our minds are thinking. With this new lens, you can practice seeing everything as a reflection.

From my observation, many women are living out a martyr story, and I am convinced that this is a major factor in why women hide behind their weight. Being a martyr is a brilliant way of hiding. You don't have to show up for yourself. You can blame others when you don't get what you want. You can live behind the mask of being a "good person". It can feel safer to give to others than to yourself. You care more about what others think of you than what you think of yourself. It feels safer to put yourself on a pedestal of being better than others because you're "doing the work", and now you can judge others

121

which keeps the connection and intimacy that you desperately desire at arm's length. You give to get and when you don't get what you expected in return, you shut your heart down. Your existence is based off of how you can convince yourself that you're worthy and lovable by helping others or through people-pleasing.

Lack of self-worth and low esteem are warped into appearing as if you got it together and are doing well in the world because you are selfless. But as one of my clients said, "being selfless is really having less of yourself." It's a tricky story because it convinces you that you are creating value, but in the meantime your energy tank is on empty and your resentment tank is overflowing.

Boundaries are the antidote for martyrdom. If you resonate with the martyr story, it is likely that your boundaries are foggy at best. You may not even realize or have the skills to gauge where the line is. You may have no clue as to what to say 'yes' to or what to say 'no' to.

One way to begin working on this is to ask yourself what it would look like if you made a conscious choice to live for yourself. What would it mean to stop going through the motions and live a life that is not based off of other people's expectations? Perhaps it's your parents' expectations that you took in while you were young, or maybe it's your partner's expectations, or your community's expectations, or society's expectations. No matter what the source is, there is no time like now to make a commitment to you. Waiting will only ensure that you will be resentful and not living the life you desire for X more days, weeks, months, years, or decades.

When you are able to create loving yet firm boundaries with your ego, it will be easier to create them in your life. And when you are able to create loving yet firm boundaries in your life, it will be easier to create them with your ego.

This connection between boundaries within yourself and with others is another mirror. There's a set of terms I learned in acupuncture school: visceral-somatic and somatic-visceral. What this means is that an internal issue such as chronic digestion issues can cause muscle tightness around the abdomen area. And muscle tightness around the abdomen area can cause digestion issues. There's no disconnect. Internal effects the external and vice versa. Micro macro. Yin yang.

You have to understand where your line is. I have my garden; you have your garden. A lot of times we're all up in another person's garden. But what about our own garden? This is what martyrs do all the time, but they have convinced themselves that they are "helping" the other person.

When you're able to see where that line is, you can redirect your attention inward. I visualize it as an arrow. Most of my life, my arrow was constantly going outward. What can I fix? What can I control? What are they thinking about me? All up in their business. Trying to be a mind reader. But when you know your boundaries and you're able to witness what's happening, you can choose to pivot and U-turn that arrow around towards yourself so you can do the only work that will actually bring you peace and happiness. Because trying to control everything in the outside world will not give it to you, and you have evidence of this over and over again. And the reality is that you will never be able to get in the other person's head and you will never be able to change anyone. So the continuation of crossing these boundaries is pure insanity, and I did this for most of my life.

BOUNDARY RESEARCH RITUAL

This is an exercise to cultivate your self-integrity. You will notice that it will activate entry points and you will have many opportunities to do the work as a result.

Create a container where you will honor your 'yes' and your 'no'. A container is similar to creating a structure with "rules". It supports your research by creating a safe space. First decide on a time period; you can do a week, a month, a year, or whatever you like. I did it for a few months and then I never stopped because it felt so good to honor myself. Decide if you are going to focus on a certain area of your life or all areas. And create any other "rules" that feel good to you.

Anytime someone asks you for something, or for you to do something, STOP, and ask yourself, "Do I desire to do this?" and let your body answer for you. Most of the time you will know the answer right away. You won't need your logical brain for this exercise. The first answer that pops up is your answer. And if you're not a big YES, then you're a no.

Now, if you're not clear about your answer or if you feel uncomfortable telling the truth you're your own answer. Let the requestor know that you will get back to them with an answer when you have had some time to consider the request. Give yourself the time to check in with yourself so that you don't feel the pressure to answer right away. People who lack boundaries, who are afraid to say no, will often feel compelled to answer a request right away. Take your time. No one will die.

If the answer is a no. Just respond with a, "no, thank you.". No need to give any excuses. It's your life, time, and energy and you get to choose what you want to do with it, without having to explain to anyone. It will feel very uncomfortable for a while but then you'll start to notice a sense of liberation. No more being a slave to your people-pleasing anymore. Notice if you're wanting to fluff up your response. You will start to see very quickly and clearly how much you have lacked boundaries and went along just because.

The great part about this is if you're a yes, you will really enjoy it and be fully present. You will start to notice all of the things that you have been saying yes to that took up so much of your time.

Also, take sure, ok, or fine out of your vocabulary when it comes to these situations. Those words ooze lack of ownership to what you want. Are you a yes or a no?

BODY BELIEFS

Limiting beliefs about our body can be covert or overt, whether the beliefs come from social media or as a result of experiencing sexual abuse or assault. The covert version is like an insidious virus. Many women have the same limiting belief – that they should be thin in order to be attractive or sexy. There are

125

so many external sources that drill this false message into our heads that we may not even realize it. Over time, these limiting belief can be like a virus and make us sick with body shame and self-hate.

One of my clients realized that she had been obsessed with releasing weight since she was a little girl because she wanted to be like the "skinny girls." She was tall and healthy, but always thought she was fat. She felt different from her peers and from the portrayal of women in the media. Feeling like an "outsider" impacts people in different ways.

It didn't help that her mother also wanted to be thin. Limiting beliefs are passed down from generation to generation until someone decides to do things differently by questioning their beliefs. Now looking back at her photos, she realizes that she wasn't fat at all, but she was convinced back then that she was. Her body dysmorphia and body shame seeds were planted when she was eight years old. From all of the feedback I've received from women, this is a very common covert belief that has made its way into the masses.

On the other hand, when a woman is sexually assaulted, it's a very overt cause of her body shame beliefs. This usually happens if she feels responsible for the abuse even though it was never her fault. Another reason is that the assault was a legit reason to hide and create body armor. She took the clear information that was given to her from her experience and made a direct correlation to how she feels about her body.

Limiting beliefs don't discriminate. Whether covert or overt, they have an impact, and if that belief lives in someone's psyche for years with no intervention, the belief will feed off of them and grow like a parasite.

THE SABOTEUR

When I started gaining more consciousness around my upper limits and my sabotaging behaviors, I started to character-ize my saboteur in order to create a clear line of distinction between who I really am versus whast my ego was trying to desperately convince me I was, because as I got to know my ego, I saw that my saboteur was really the fearful, young parts of me that didn't receive the love and attention I needed as a child, the part of me that was in survival mode and just wanted protection, at all cost. As I got to know her, an image appeared of my eight-year-old self.

She was adorable and a terror at the same time. She was running amok and would be spying on me from around the corner, just waiting for the right time to attack. I saw this inno-cent, little, fearful girl who knew no better, so I decided to be the adult and love her as she was. I put her at the kid's table with a blankie and her friends. She felt safe there. So, every time she would act out, I would find a way to soothe her and give her a sense of safety. Sometimes, it was tucking her in a cozy bed with stuffed animals. Other times, I would cud-dle her. Immediately, her nervous system would relax, which meant that my nervous system relaxed.

It was effective because I was able to separate her from me. I could see how her fear was the culprit, not her. I was able to see her with a compassionate heart.

It's not about blocking out the ego or thoughts, it's about knowing that it's just what the ego does. It's not personal. It's how we're wired as humans. Once you stop taking it personally, you can look at it from a distance. You see that you have the power in the dynamic, and you practice using it in your everyday life.

TANTRUM LOVE RITUAL

Start by observing your most repeated, most negative thoughts, the ones that are like a broken record. Then picture yourself as a child when you first started to feel insecure or fearful. Connect with her. What is she wearing? What is her facial expression? What is she feeling?

Imagine her having a tantrum while screaming those repetitive, broken-record, thoughts. Look at her through motherly, compassionate eyes. Can you see that she is in pain and that she just needs love? Can you open up your heart to her? Now create a scene where you are loving her. What would you have wanted as a child? What is she wanting? Give her the love and attention that soothes her. Let her nervous system relax.

When you both feel complete, take a moment to tell her you love her and appreciate her just as she is.

QUESTIONING AND VISUALIZING

Perhaps you are a very curious person already, but do you limit your questions to areas that you feel confident and comfortable in already? Are you asking questions that stem from a limiting belief? What would happen if you started asking questions that were completely out of the box?

One of my participants knew that she had been carrying around a martyr story. She knew it inside out and outside in. Her awareness was off the charts, but she still carried this martyr story like a badge of honor. The problem was that she was asking herself the wrong questions over and over again, which lead her to continue the cycle of suffering. It wasn't until she asked herself, "If I dared to do things differently, what would that look like?", that her life began to change dramatically. She was able to go to exercises classes where before she felt guilty for leaving her kids with a nanny. She was able to ask her husband for the type of sensual touch she desired for the first time after being together for twenty years.

Curiosity isn't just about asking interesting questions, although that's a game-changing tool. You must also look at life with awe; see the world and people as they really are: fascinating.

So much of the time, we are making statements as if they are facts instead of asking questions. When we are able to ask questions instead, it can shift our minds from tunnel vision to seeing other options and perspectives. And if you add the power of visualization, you have a powerful combination to rewire your brain. Neuroplasticity is a real thing but it can't happen if you don't practice. If you don't practice, your mind continues down the same path it's always gone down. It's like the movie Groundhogs Day. Most people use imagination in a way that is of disservice to themselves and others, instead of constructive. For example, they will envision all of the awful things that have happened over and over again instead of envisioning the possibilities.

The first issue is that people are usually asking the wrong questions because they are focused on asking "why?". 'Why?' has a tendency to be a huge distraction and creates a rabbit hole of questioning in the wrong direction. 'Why?' is all about the past and has you ruminating about all of your woes, which is different than feeling emotions that arise from an entry point activation. Asking 'why?' over and over is like a cat chasing their tail. It will just have you spinning in the same spot. The most potent questions are the ones that open your mind to what's possible for you in areas you haven't considered before. Your brain gets to make new connections when this happens and you open up to other ways of being because you're experiencing it through the power of visualization and feeling it as if you were there. If you never see what's possible then you can't know it's available to you. Just like if you'd never heard of chocolate, you would never crave it.

THE TWO VERSIONS OF YOU RITUAL

- *Here's a list of powerful questions you can use to do this ritual or you can create your own question. Ask the question in connection with a specific situation happening in your current life.*
- *How would life look and feel if I dared to do things I desired?*
- *What would happen if I let go of this resentment? How would I feel? How would life be different?*

- *How would life change if I stopped putting everyone else before me? How would I feel?*
- *What would happen if I trusted the Universe?*
- *How would life be for me if I stopped hiding?*
- *How would life feel if I released my fear fat suit?*
- *How would life be different if I chose me first?*
- *How would I feel, be, or treat myself and others if I didn't believe this thought or belief?*
- *What if I choose to see this situation differently?*

Sit in a private and quiet place and close your eyes. Take three deeps breaths to get into this present moment and your body. Imagine two identical images of you next to each other. The one on the left is the current you who is suffering in a current situation and the one on the right is the future you who is able to see other possibilities. The idea is that the left version of you is how you've lived your life with a certain belief that has created suffering and the right version of you is the you who doesn't believe the belief that has created suffering.

Ask yourself one of the questions above in the negative aspect to the left version of you and then in the positive aspect to the right version of you. Ask one question at a time for each version. For example: The first question "How would life look and feel if I dared to do things I desired? In the negative is "How would life look and feel when I don't dare to do things I desire?"

Allow each version of you to feel all of the emotions that arise when asked the question. When you ask the question to yourself, images will arise. Allow them to come up on their own and explore what's happening with curiosity.

Now compare the two: Visualize how different their lives are from each other and how different they feel. Let yourself visualize your life playing out as if it were a movie and you're the star actor. Don't force the images. Take it in and notice how you are the one who's in control over your beliefs and how they impact your life.

When you feel complete, take three deeps breaths to reconnect with your body. Take a moment to thank the Universe, your ancestors, and loved ones on the other side for all of their love, holding, and guidance. And then slowly open your eyes. Journal about your experience so you can digest what just happened. Insights, images, words, feelings, memories. Write freely without too much thought. Let your hands do the writing. Then take your time transitioning into what you need to do next.

The beauty of this mediation is that you get to see how much power and control you have in your life, that you can say 'no' to your ego whenever you choose. It becomes clearer that you need to practice focusing your attention and choosing something different than what you've been habitually thinking and believing.

Also, remember to consider doing *The Work* by Byron Katie. Her system uses four simple questions and a turn around process to help you with your belief inquiry.

"When you start sacrificing yourself for other people, you make them a thief, because they are stealing from you what you need and they don't even know it."
— Iyanla Vanzant

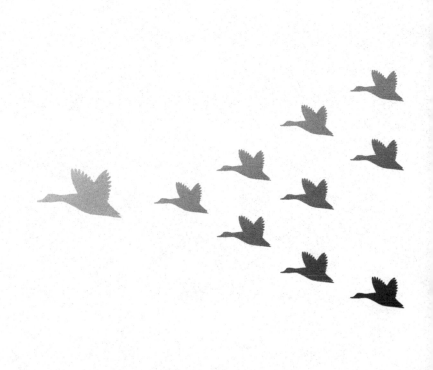

CHAPTER 8

THE BODY KNOWS
(THE PHYSICAL REALM)

*"There is more wisdom in your body than in
your deepest philosophies."*
— Friedrich Nietzche

It's a sacred act to love your body, but what does loving your body mean exactly? It means approving of how you look, listening to what it is communicating with you, trusting what it is telling you, and taking care of it accordingly - and your body will take care of you in return.

Releasing weight is a spiritual practice, and for women who have done tons of emotional and spiritual work, it's also the final frontier. This practice of being present in your body is deeply spiritual because if you are unable to love and care for your temple in a way that is, honoring its perfection, you are telling the ultimate creator, source energy, that you don't trust it, the laws of nature, or yourself.

I have found from all of my explorations in the healing realms that this journey of releasing weight was the most profound because it was my final frontier and required such cultivation of intimacy with myself. The work must be done in all the realms, or else the weight release won't stick.

I used to hate that I was overweight because it reminded me of the imbalance within myself. I was tired all of the time and didn't have the energy to do anything that I wanted to do. I was an isolated couch potato who lived in a fantasy land of wishing and hoping that my desires would magically come to me but I didn't want to do anything to go after them. Magical thinking can take over your life if you let it. I just wanted the weight off, I didn't want to do the work in order to make it happen. But now, I realize that my weight-releasing journey was a gift.

This journey has given me the opportunity to align with the divine in a way that I don't know if I would have been able to without it. If we are able to alchemize our deepest fears and pains and use them to transform ourselves, our connection to source energy grows, and from there, anything is possible.

That possibility comes from your newly cultivated intuition. As you do this work, your intuition will get clearer and louder. You will be tapped into a power that is all-knowing. There will be a sense of peace that comes from this level of trust and surrender. You will be able to connect to the unseen world.

Since my traumas, I became a prisoner in my body. I was disconnected from it to the point of disassociation. It became a way of being which I thought was normal. I had no idea that I was living outside of my body. I only had clues like when I had sex and would notice myself checking out and I would have to consciously bring myself back to the present. I would also dissociate when I felt anxious in new social settings. I didn't know I was so disconnected from my body because, for me, this had become my normal. When you live a certain way for most of your life, you may not know what's missing. It wasn't until I started doing embodiment practices that I started to connect in palpable ways with my body.

Cultivating a deeper level of connection with your body begins with feeling the sensations that live inside of you. I view sensations as little fairies that live in me. They are potent entry points into a magical land of discovery and healing. Just like all entry points, sensations guide you into unconscious spaces that store information that can set you free.

IDENTIFYING SENSATIONS

I always tell my patients to listen to what their body is telling them, but what does that mean exactly? How do you know what your body is trying to tell you if you don't even have a relationship with it? The intention of this chapter is for you to develop an intimate relationship with your body so you can listen to its infinite wisdom. But first you need to practice feeling. Just like when you connect with your emotional feelings, you will practice feeling sensations in the body. That's one of the reasons why I love acupuncture – it helps you to connect with your body by way of sensations. During an acupuncture session a client can feel a range of sensations such as: throbbing, heaviness, waves of energy flowing through the body, and electricity. Identifying and feeling sensations is like learning a new language, the language of your body, and this takes some practice.

In the beginning, what often happens is that people automatically judge sensations to mean something that they have been conditioned to believe. For example, you may have adopted the belief that a racing heart means you are anxious, but it could mean you are excited. We tend to interpret our sensations through our mind and then act on them based on our initial and pre-conditioned interpretations. Instead, what would happen if you just felt the sensation without making any assumptions of what it meant? This is called mindfulness. It's the same practice that you've been practicing with your emotions and your thoughts, and now you're doing it with your body.

BODY SCAN RITUAL

Use this ritual whether you feel an intense sensation like a sharp pain or when you are feeling no sensations at all and would like to explore getting in touch with some.

Sit down in a private and quiet space. Take three deeps breaths and connect with your body. Put your attention on your toes and see if you feel any sensations and slowly move up your body, one body part at a time until you get to the top of your head.

Go slowly so you can connect with any sensations.

If you feel a sensation, focus your attention on it.

Feel it without trying to change it or control it. Just be with it. It may dissipate or it may not. It may move or it may not. It may change to a different quality or temperature or it may not. Just be with it. And then move to the next body part.

You may experience images spontaneously arising. You may hear a message. You may notice a particular feeling or you may not. If you do, or even if you don't, try to stay curious.

If, like a sled, the sensation wants to guide you to another sensation or memory, go with it. If memories or emotions arise, simply be with them. Hold space for yourself as described in the emotional realm chapter.

You can also ask the sensation a question like, "what do you want me to know?". And just let the answer arise. See what your body wants to tell you. If it doesn't have a message, that's ok. You are cultivating a relationship with your body in a new way. Just like when connecting with a new friend or lover, it takes time to feel comfortable and safe to open up. Be loving and kind to your body.

When you feel complete, take three deeps breaths to reconnect with your body. Take a moment to thank the Universe, your ancestors, and loved ones on the other side for all of their love, holding, and guidance. And then slowly open your eyes. Journal about your experience so you can digest what just happened. Insights, images, words, feelings, memories. Write freely without too much thought. Let your hands do the writing. Then take your time transitioning into what you need to do next.

Just like with your emotions and your thoughts, you will now give your body space to express itself, and all you need to do is listen and feel. The act of giving your body space to feel without putting your thoughts onto it will actually be the thing that allows your relationship with it to cultivate over time.

Begin by sitting in quiet and stillness and do a body scan. Start by putting your attention on your feet, feel them, and then move your attention up your body slowly up your legs, hips, torso, arms, neck, head. Every area of your body has a voice. Be curious and see if you feel something.

After a time, you will be able to feel sensations while on the move, around a bunch of people; wherever and whenever you like. It's all about cultivating your attention. As you get more in tune with your sensations, it will be easier to feel sensations in situations where you couldn't before.

Whether you have intense sensations or not, it's a great practice to pay attention to them throughout the day. Doing check-ins will shift your relationship with your body. You can sit at your desk at work, close your eyes, start your body scan, and take note of what you're feeling. Perhaps your toes feel cold; there's some subtle tingling in your thighs; your low back feels tight and achy; your stomach feels warm; your right index fingertip has an electric sensation; your chest feels heavy; and your forehead is achy.

This is not uncommon to have all these different sensations happening at one time. It takes time and practice to identify them and learn how to express these sensations into words.

Sensations are complex and are made up of different aspects. Here's a guideline that will help you to identify them and give language to them:

- Intensity: very subtle to very extreme and everything in between.
- Qualities: temperature-based (hot, warm, cold), electricity, tingles, sharpness, aches, heaviness, burning, pinching, tight, soft, numbness, etc.
- Temperature: cold, warm, hot, chilly
- Duration: range from a quick moment to long-lasting.
- Location: anywhere in the body.

Sensations can give us messages about what our physical and emotional bodies need. They are a guide if we let them be. Once you practice listening to your body, you will eventually be able to have a conversation with it. You will learn to interpret the sensations with your intuition, not your mind.

A week after I broke up with my ex, I had an accident that tore my shoulder labrum. It was the most intense sensation I had ever experienced. After the initial frustration that this happened, I got clear that it happened because I was feeling so guilty because of my martyrdom story and that I was subconsciously punishing myself. But the thing is, I used this high-intensity sharp sensation in my shoulder to guide me through my emotional healing process and my weight-releasing process.

I was forced to slow down because if I didn't, I would feel everything intensely. I had to take exquisite care of myself so

I could heal. I had to put all of the attention on self-care versus my guilt. The pain became my daily moment-to-moment meditation. It kept bringing me back to my body over and over. It was such a gift.

It's also a reminder that injuries don't need to be a roadblock in our weight-releasing journey because this is the time when I released forty pounds. So, no excuses when it comes to injuries. I chose exercises that didn't bother my arm like jogging and jumping on my trampoline. If the desire is there, anything is possible.

Most of the time, people are annoyed by the sensations in their bodies and just want to get rid of them. You have a stomachache, and you just take medicine to get rid of the discomfort, but did you take a moment to ask your stomach what it needs? What's the underlying root issue that needs attention here? Band-Aids only last so long. What if we asked what medicine we really need right now and were able to listen to what our bodies tell us?

I have had many powerful experiences where a sensation has brought me deeper into healing. I recall a specific moment during another breakup: I was triggered in this particular moment and thought that I was being used for sex. I went home, laid in my bed, and all of a sudden, I felt a strong ache in my chest, and my heart started beating faster. Perhaps someone else would have labeled it anxiety and from that label would have actually created an anxiety attack. But I was clear that it was just sensation, and it was trying to tell me something.

I closed my eyes and allowed myself to sink into it. Then all of a sudden, the sensation took me to a memory of my first rape. I was brought back to the exact moment where he was penetrating me. I looked in his eyes and felt the pain inside of him. I was overcome by compassion for this person who had hurt me. Then the sensation moved down to my lower abdomen, feeling heavy and thick. I was then brought to a recent memory of the man I had just broken up with and was able to feel that same level of compassion for him, even though just moments before, I was categorizing him as a perpetrator. It felt like a trip, but I was completely sober.

This is what's possible when we feel. Sensations are like sleds. They can lead us to these powerful entry points of healing if you surrender to them.

THE YANG PORTAL

CHAPTER 9

TURN YOUR BODY ON

*"Within my body are all the sacred places of the world,
and the most profound pilgrimage I can ever make is
within my own body."*
— Saraha

DANCING

Dancing is a surefire way of getting in your body and turning on. If you are stuck in your head and need a reset, put on your favorite jams and let the music move you. I'm guessing pretty much everyone has experienced the power of dancing. Music has such a powerful effect on your emotional state, imagine what happens when you pair it with dancing like there's no tomorrow, and when you let your moves be full of heart.

You can dance every morning as soon as you wake up to get your juices moving, or you can dance once every hour while at work. Perhaps you're doing your taxes and need to get turned on to keep you from procrastinating. That's what I did. I literally filed for an extension every year for as long as I could remember, but when I used dancing as a tool to get turned on, I was able to file my taxes not only on time, but early! Miracles happen when we are tapped into the electricity that is available to us at any moment; even tax miracles!

Add a mirror to get even more connected to yourself. Witness your joy and love bursting out of you and get even more turned on. You have this amazing body that you were born into and it's here to live life and to be in pleasure. Flirt with yourself. Dance sensually. Dance like a wild woman. However your body wants to move, do it.

DANCING RITUAL

Turn on whatever song that makes you feel whatever emotion you're feeling or desire to feel. And dance like no one's watching. Get into it. Feel your energy rise as you let any heaviness or worries that are present wash away. Check yourself out in the mirror. Smile at yourself. Circle those hips! However your body wants to move, just do it. She knows what she wants so follow her lead. Feel the elation and electricity rise. This is you in all of your expressive glory. Don't hold back. This moment is all for you. Feel the turn-on that lives in you. You were made for this.

When you feel complete, take a moment to thank your beautiful body, your loved ones on the other side, and your higher power for holding space for this alchemical journey.

MIRROR WORK

Another way of cultivating a loving and intimate relationship with your body is to see the beauty of it, as it is. Do you ever look at yourself naked in a full-length mirror? Seeing yourself exactly as you are, with no judgment, is a game-changer.

When we transform what was once negative in our minds to something beautiful, anything is possible. Our bodies truly become a work of art, whether we are overweight or not. Mirror work is powerful because you get to be with yourself in a way that is open and connected. Normally when we look in the mirror, it's prepping how we want to be seen in the world like when we do our make-up or hair or even practical reasons, like flossing our teeth. But how often do you look at yourself to say how much you love you or tell yourself how beautiful you are? Mirror work allows us to see us as we are and learn full acceptance, approval, and love of self.

MIRROR WORK RITUAL

Start by eye-gazing with yourself close to the mirror. Connect with yourself. Look at yourself as if you were your lover, with loving, affectionate eyes. Look so deeply that you can feel your own soul.

Once you feel that loving connection, step back and take a look at your entire body, naked in all of its glory. You may feel twinges of judgments or full-on self-hatred. Whatever arises is okay. Just notice what your thoughts are and make a note of it. Take a deep breath and then look at yourself again with soft eyes (that means to relax your eyes so they're kind of in a dreamy state, like half-way closed).

Look at the part of your body that you love the most and gaze at it with affection. Tell yourself, in your mind or out loud, how much you love it and thank it for all it has done for you while touching it lovingly. If it's your legs, you can say something like, "I love you. Thank you for being so strong, keeping me rooted, and taking me wherever I've needed to go."

Then go to a part of your body you have judgments about. Still with a soft, loving gaze, touch it and caress it while you thank it and tell it you love it. If it's your stomach, you could say, "I love you. Thank you for protecting my sex organs all these years. I needed this layer of fat to feel safe, and I appreciate you for honoring my need for safety."

Make sure to include scars, stretch marks, and cellulite on your list of things to put loving attention on. This will impact you more than you can ever imagine.

If you can't find any gratitude yet, just caress it with love. Then try next time to find the words. Start off with one part you love and one part you don't love. Then you can increase these based on how you feel. I recommend doing this daily for about five to ten minutes first thing in the morning or before bed.

When you feel complete, take a moment to thank your reflection, your loved ones on the other side, and your higher power for holding space for this transformative experience.

After I lost forty pounds, I noticed that I had new stretch marks on my butt, calves, breasts, and upper arms. At first, I freaked and had a moment of disappointment and judgment. My vision of what I thought I wanted disappeared just like that. But as I've shared, entry point activations are gifts because they open the portal into healing. So I used this opportunity to love myself even more.

I did mirror work on my stretch marks every day for a few days, and there was a moment when I looked at them and felt a deep love for them when I saw an image of the rings on a tree. Each ring around a tree represents a year of existence. They are growth rings. I felt this profound sense of love for my growth marks and for how my body has gone through so much over the years and still stood there with so much power and vitality. My growth marks are now an indication of my emotional maturity and physical strength to move through challenging times in my life, not an indication of failure.

SELF-PLEASURE

I also recommend self-pleasuring as often as you can, not only touching your erogenous zones but also all areas of your body. Perhaps your tummy likes being held, or maybe your thigh likes to be caressed, or perhaps your ear likes a little pinch. Get to know what feels good to you. What sensations do you like? What sensations do you not? Put attention on the parts that you tend to ignore. Rub them, caress them, stroke them.

Your body has been ignored and shamed long enough. You must take a radical step if you want radical self-love. Even if you feel like you're faking it at first, do it anyway, no matter what your ego tries to tell you. Your resistance will demand that you do something else more important, like Netflix. Or perhaps you'll have an urge to emotionally eat in that very moment. These are all perfect because they are signals giving you information, which is telling you about your resistance. Maybe you are afraid and want to check out, but resistances usually arise when we are close to an opening or a breakthrough.

SELF-PLEASURE RITUAL

Create space to be present with yourself, whether in your bedroom, in your office, on the train. Wherever you are, let your fingers and hands explore your body. If in a public space, perhaps using the tip of your finger to slide gently along the top of your hand. If in private, feel free to be as naked or as clothed as you desire.

Be curious and take your time. Go slowly and fully receive your touch.

Touch a spot on your body that you've never put attention on or touch a spot that you have put attention on but now touch it in a new way. How does it feel to the spot being touched? How does it feel to the part doing the touching? Take in this moment and feel how the subtle sensations are turning your body on. Soak in the juiciness that is you. Connect with the deliciousness of your body.

When you feel complete, take a moment to thank your body, your loved ones on the other side, and your higher power for holding space for this sensual experience.

SWEET TALK

How many times have you done the opposite of sweet-talking to yourself? Are you downright mean to yourself about your body? Is it a constant stream of subtle negative internal comments you make to yourself? I dare you to flip this script and start talking to yourself in the loving way that a lover would. Whisper sweet nothings as you caress your soft skin. Use a tone that is generous and loving, and do it often.

Whenever you notice yourself saying unkind things to yourself, it's the perfect time to sweet talk yourself. Or try sweet talking to yourself when you're feeling stressed. Or sweet talk for no other reason than that you just want to love on yourself. You don't even have to have a reason. Do it because it feels good. You deserve to be talked to with kindness, appreciation, and love. Have you ever considered that when you overeat sweet foods, that what you really might be craving is another kind of sweetness altogether? Like many of the practices in this book, sweet-talk may feel weird or uncomfortable at first, but I believe that as you continue to practice, you will find yourself enjoying the playfulness and the pleasure that ensues. Sweet talk will start to feel like home, like you may even exclaim, "How have I not done this all of my life?"

SWEET TALK RITUAL

While looking in a mirror with soft eyes, tell yourself how amazing you are. Believe it. Tell yourself that you are beautiful, lovable, sexy, or kind. Tell yourself how proud you are of yourself. Whatever you say, say it with love and a generous heart. And reciprocate that love by receiving it with an open heart.

This is a moment to connect with the perfection of who you are while allowing yourself to feel your spirit And please know: you are your own best friend. You have your own back.

This ritual can be as long or as short as you like. You can say one sweet sentence or you can go on and on about how amazing, adorable, and precious you are for as long as you desire. The most important part is not the length of the ritual, but to receive the words graciously.

When you feel complete, take a moment to thank yourself, your loved ones on the other side, and your higher power for holding space for this self-love fest.

As you cultivate this new relationship with your body via your sensations, mirror work, self-pleasure, and sweet-talking, you will start to notice both subtle and big shifts. You'll notice that it starts to get easier to look at yourself in a loving way. You'll genuinely feel gratitude for certain parts of your body that you completely hated before. You'll notice that you're not saying as many judgmental things to yourself about your body. You'll notice that you'll want to look at yourself in the mirror more because it feels good to connect with yourself. You'll be enraptured by you and how sexy and sensual you are! Let the momentum take a hold of you and run with it.

You'll eventually get to a place where your limited definition of beauty that was dictated by society or your family is now expanding into a new definition, one that is coming from inside of you, from a feeling born in your body versus a false idea of perfection. You will find yourself living in a dream state, but it's based in reality. You don't have to live up to a false standard anymore. You can create your own standard that's based on your connection with the truths that live within you. They were just covered with shame, but once the shame releases, you will be able to identify those truths based on love that has been living inside of you since you were born.

We all were born with the knowledge that we are perfect as we are. We've just had layers upon layers of lies implanted in us. I love that gemstones are quite breathtaking, even when they're not perfect. Even the most beautiful diamond has imperfections, and that's what makes it uniquely perfect. Do you really want to look like someone else? We are not meant to be clones. We are human and we are special in our own ways and that not only includes our personalities but our appearances too. I want to encourage you to find the beauty in who you are. Own it. Get turned-on by it, really start to shine.

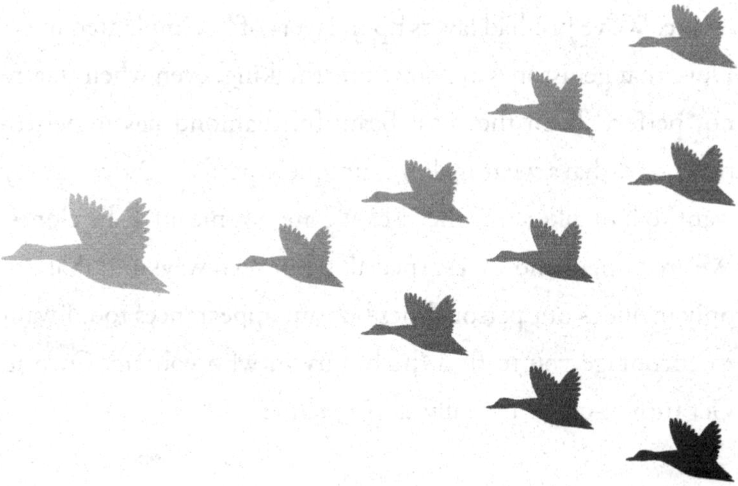

CHAPTER 10

SLEEP, FOOD AND EXERCISE... OH MY!

"Your body is a temple but only if you treat it as one."
— Astrid Alauda

As you've learned, spiritual bypassing causes backed-up emotions in the body which can lead to illness, pain, etc. But what happens when we emotionally bypass our physical needs? It's not talked about in the self-development community, but it's something I've personally experienced in the past, and I see many others doing the same. It's easy to use "doing the emotional or spiritual work" as an excuse to not do the physical work. When we ignore one or more of the realms, an imbalance is created. In some healing communities, there is a hierarchy, and the physical realm is on the bottom.

In my experience coming from a history of putting all of my attention on the emotional and spiritual and pretty much avoiding the mental and physical for most of my life, I can tell you that each realm is equal because they rely on each other and impact each other, just as yin and yang do. They have different qualities, unique to them, but each is just as important as the other.

Being healthy is the key here and as a result of being healthy, your body will become the appropriate size for you. This isn't about chasing a weight. It's about taking exquisite care of yourself in all ways, including your health. It's true what they say, that health is wealth. If you don't have your health, the most extreme result is that you will die. The other side is that you will have a low quality of life, of exhaustion, and no energy to create the life you desire. In a sense, you may feel like the walking dead because one day falls into the next and there's no sense of purpose or connection to yourself. Being healthy is the priority in this chapter. When you are healthy, you feel alive and are ready to take on the world and live with passion.

CULTIVATING GOOD SLEEP HABITS

I am starting with sleep because it's something that people have an idea of how important it is but don't prioritize it because they don't *really* know how important it is.

Quality sleep not only allows your body to recover and restore after a workout; it is a key ingredient in releasing weight but also heals every other aspect of you – emotional, mental, and physical. If you don't get quality sleep, your cortisol hormone can elevate which can cause weight gain, high blood pressure, muscle weakness, stress, etc.

Unrestful sleep has also been known to cause more sugar, carbohydrate, and caffeine cravings. If the body is exhausted, it needs something external to give it energy. But here is the thing, our energy should come from a healthy internal state that is sourced by healthy nutrients for the mind and body and a state of being. If it's not, it's a false sense of energy that covers up the root issues.

The interesting part that I have observed in my acupuncture practice is that stress is usually the cause of unrestful sleep. Most people tend to go to bed too late because they can't shut their minds off (stress) or they can't stop looking at screens, like TVs, computers, or phones (avoiding stress). Or they are eating or drinking too much alcohol too often or too late (numbing stress). Or they aren't moving their body (stress build-up). Or they have been drinking coffee all day because they're trying to hit a work deadline (stress).

Just because you get eight hours of sleep doesn't mean you are getting the quality sleep your mind and body need. Are you tossing and turning or waking up in the middle of the night? Do you wake up feeling tired? Do you need coffee or caffeine to get your day started? If so, then you're not getting quality sleep.

Here's some ways that you can get better sleep:

- Daily meditation.
- Consistent exercise.
- Go to bed by 11pm.
- More time in nature.

- Integrate a nighttime ritual (discussed in the next chapter).
- Check if your blood values are off and get the minerals and vitamins you need.
- Decrease sugar, carbs, caffeine and alcohol (especially in the late afternoon/evening).
- Do the entry point rituals.

INTUITIVE EATING

Intuitive eating is the remedy for emotional eating. When you emotionally eat, you have a clear indicator that you are off-balance somewhere and you're probably not fully listening to your inner wisdom, feelings, and sensations. It is important to build your intuitive muscles in this process. Doing so will serve you, not only with releasing weight, but in all areas of your life. This starts now with trusting what your body is telling you, day to day, moment by moment.

Food is necessary to maintain our life, literally. But we can also be alive but not living. I'm always amazed at how people are alive but never drink water and consume a large part of their meals as processed foods. If this is you, ask yourself if you really want a life where you feel energized, and if you do, are you ready to really live one?

I ask these questions because, when you feel revitalized, it feels like living on purpose. But, it's hard to feel this fully when you are unhealthy. Being healthy doesn't equal being skinny either, but it does mean that you are making conscious and informed decisions. Are you connected to your food? Do you know where your food is coming from? Do you look at the ingredients that you're ingesting? Get curious about what you are putting in your body and the chemical effects it has. It's quite fascinating actually. The human body is beyond miraculous, and we take it for granted most of the time.

My goal isn't to tell you exactly what to eat. I will make suggestions, but this path is not a diet. Everyone has a different constitution and preferences. When we put food into our bodies without being conscious and mindful, we can get into dangerous territory, especially when we have a history of emotional eating. I'm not saying to never eat sugar, carbs, etc. I would never say that! I am a foodie and will always have my fair share of pasta, fried chicken, and ice cream. But making conscious choices versus unconscious choices are two very different things.

This is where the practice of witnessing yourself comes into play. When it comes to food, staying present within yourself is the key. Checking in and asking yourself radically honest questions will help you stay true to your desire of releasing weight and feeling good while doing it.

I found out during my weight-releasing journey that I wasn't as hungry as I always thought I was. Before I started paying attention, I was in a habitual cycle of eating all the time without awareness. I would just put things in my mouth without thinking about it. I didn't really connect with how and what I was eating or how foods made me physically feel because I was living with a baseline of feeling yucky to begin with. I didn't know that I could feel so good, energized, and strong in my body because I never gave myself the opportunity to experience anything like that.

Give yourself permission to experiment with listening to your body and following through with what it tells you. Play with asking yourself, "What would happen when I eat this? Or that?" Create a container to research what feels good and what doesn't. Learn when you're really hungry and when you're not, when you're eating because you're stressed or when you're bored. If you've been an emotional eater all your life, like me, it will take time and practice. But the key is to play with it. Be curious.

I recommend creating a food awareness section in your Self Journal (explained in the next chapter) as you get to know yourself better in these ways. This is not to track calories! I don't believe in that. More so, it's to create a higher level of awareness when it comes to food or any habits you're shifting. Write down all that you've observed in your research on a daily basis.

For example, this could be an entry: "I thought I was hungry this afternoon. I ended up eating some toast with butter. It wasn't satisfying at all. I still felt 'hungry' even though I wasn't really hungry. Now looking back, I realize I wasn't hungry in the first place. I was feeling lonely. I just wanted to feel connected to something or someone." The nugget here is that there's a new awareness of what hunger is and isn't. I now have a body memory of that moment, of when I thought I was hungry but really wasn't. I can use that memory anytime in the future when that similar feeling arises. This is redefining your conditioned habits around food, one experience at a time. With time and practice, you will create a "catalog" of these body memories that you can also tap into for guidance.

MINDFUL EATING RITUAL

Before you eat, send loving energy to your food. Thank it for the nourishment it will provide you. Take a bite and chew. Pay attention to the taste and textures and chew more slowly. Enjoy every bite and savor it. You may want to put your utensil down in between every bit to bring more presence to the experience. Be aware of your emotional state. Do you have an urge to eat faster? Watch your thoughts. Is your mind drifting to you to do list or is it present with your experience of your meal? Take your time and let your level of hunger catch up with you naturally. But mostly importantly, enjoy the act of eating, of taking in nourishment and sustenance.

When you are finished eating, take a moment to thank your food, yourself, your loved ones on the other side, and your higher power for holding space for this deliciously mindful experience.

There are hunger hormones in our bloodstream that communicate with our brain and send a signal when we are hungry and full. The thing is that it takes about twenty minutes to receive the full signal. So if you're wolfing down food, you will most definitely overeat and feel stuffed. But the great news is that this is avoidable if you eat mindfully. Take your time, and give your internal body systems a chance to guide you. Plus, food tastes so much better when we take our time.

Most people who have struggled with overeating won't stop eating until they feel uncomfortably full. But again, it's been such a habit that it feels normal to be that full. Try experimenting with how it feels to eat until you feel satisfied. That means your stomach feels comfortable, and you don't feel hungry anymore. Ask yourself, "Am I wanting to continue eating because my body or my mind is telling me to?" Then wait for the answer. If you pause and give yourself the space and time to be present while both preparing and also while eating your meals, you will have a better chance of *not* overeating.

If you are craving something that is outside of the structure you have designed for yourself, ask yourself why. You may already be clear that you want to emotionally eat and if that's the case, take out your journal and start writing. Your prompt is: "I want to eat _____ because I am feeling _____." Let yourself feel the emotions that are there and question any beliefs that are showing up.

If you still want to eat the thing, then you have three options.

- Eat it and enjoy it with all of your being by releasing the guilt.
- Find another food that is comparable, but healthier (i.e., yogurt instead of ice cream) and notice if that does the trick.
- Reach out and connect with someone because you may want to eat because what you're really needing instead is support and connection.

As a guideline, do not keep junk food in your home. Having easy access to foods that are not healthy for you will possibly tempt you in moments when you are feeling emotionally over-whelmed. This doesn't mean you can't ever eat them; it simply means that you are creating good boundaries with yourself to prevent sabotage.

Since the foundation of my teachings is based on yin and yang, it's important to allow flow (intuitive eating) and also create structure (intermittent fasting). Staying in tune with this balance will create a powerful and divine environment for you to powerfully shift your relationship with food and eating.

INTERMITTENT FASTING

I'm such a geek when it comes to the body. I research, research, research! Then I practice on myself to see what feels good to me and use that information to learn more about myself and what I need.

In my extensive research, I've learned that every time you eat, your insulin spikes, even if you eat something super healthy like kale. If you are eating throughout the day, including snacking, your insulin will spike every time. This consistent spiking of insulin can cause your body to become insulin-resistant, and as a result, your body gains weight, especially in your stomach region. Learning this kind of blew my mind!

The other part that's important to acknowledge is that we currently live in a culture that eats way too much and way too often. We have been conditioned by society to put something into our mouths at all times because somewhere along the line there was a massive lie disseminated, which told hopeful weight-releasers and really everyone for that matter, that it's healthier to eat every two to three hours. Our culture has been cultivated to live in excess and overindulgence as a way to disconnect from what's happening underneath the surface. Feeling hunger has also been skewed into a thing that needs immediate attention or else we will die. No, folks, you will not die. Hunger is not an emergency.

You will learn what levels of hunger you really have because right now, you may only have two buttons: hungry and stuffed. There's quite a spectrum in between those two states, and intermittent fasting (IF) will help you discover the full range.

The way intermittent fasting works is that everyday you have a fasting period and an eating period. These can be in different ratios, but what has worked well for me is a daily sixteen-hour fasting period followed by an eight-hour eating period. You can choose the time of the day that works best for you. I prefer having my first meal around noon, my second meal around 4 p.m., and my last around 8 p.m.

I recommend starting with a twelve-hour period of fasting and a twelve-hour eating period. Over the course of a week or two, increase the fasting period to sixteen hours.

Since insulin spikes every time you eat, I recommend no snacking and eating meals every four hours. This means that you'll need to add more healthy fats in your diet; avocados, nuts, olive oil, and ghee are all great choices. Healthy fats help to sustain your hunger longer. I also recommend cutting your sugar and carbs down quite a bit because chemically they make you get hungrier faster and, more realistically, ravenous, which will make the four hours between meals torture. Believe me, I learned the hard way. Finally, it's important to drink a lot of water with electrolytes and eat plenty of veggies when you're doing IF.

For more information on intermittent fasting, watch Dr. Berg or Dr. Rhonda Patrick's YouTube videos.

When you create structure in your day for your meals, you are more apt to follow it versus saying, "Oh, I'll just wing it," and opt for takeout. So, create a plan of what you'll eat and when, but more importantly, be willing to listen to your body in the moment because she always knows best.

I have found that IF mixed with intuitive eating feels the best for me. It's the perfect balance of yin and yang. It will require you to practice tuning in to yourself within this new eating schedule. For example, I just shared with you my typical eating schedule, but that's not what I do every day. It's the structure I typically use, but there are days when I feel hungrier earlier, and so I'll have my first meal earlier. There are days when I want to eat more carbs, so I let myself eat more carbs. There are days that I only want one or two meals a day. There are other days that I have a pint of ice cream. I don't believe in being too rigid because that typically creates resentment and frustration, which can lead to sabotage, emotional eating, ultimately binging and giving up.

I fully own and celebrate how much I love food, and I will never make myself eat in a rigid way. I also know that when

I create a structure that works for me, I feel so much better. Allow days or meals where you can eat things outside of your healthier meals. This will be different for everyone. For me, I loved planning what I was going to eat during my weekdays. I made those meals really healthy, and I let myself eat more treats on the weekends. You need to get to know yourself and what your flow is. Then, you can play around with different structures to see what works for you. But within whatever structure you decide on, it's important to be kind to yourself. This isn't about being militant or overly rigid. It's about developing a more intimate relationship with yourself so you can hear your body more clearly and trust what she's telling you.

Side note: I don't call those weekend meals "cheat meals" because I'm not cheating on anything. I'm just living my life in a conscious way that feels good to me.

Truthfully, sometimes I'll fall off the horsey, and find myself in an old pattern of emotionally eating. I don't beat myself up for this because I have realistic expectations and know there will be bumps in the road. It's about the practice of doing my best, being kind to myself, exploring the emotional and mental aspects that need tending to and loving up on my body, and then choosing to recommit to the process. Then repeat!

This is a journey, people! Not a destination. I know you've heard it many times and you get it, but are you practicing it?

So, my recommendation is this: Create an intermittent fasting schedule, follow your body's innate wisdom, and you are well on your way to feeling alive in your body! In my own experience of doing IF, I experienced a huge increase in energy, easy weight release, better sleep, a clearer mind, a better mood, and a higher level of connection with my body. Now let's move onto to exercise!

EXERCISE

The thing that I dreaded doing all my life has become something I crave now. I am still pinching myself when I think about how much I enjoy working out and have a relatively easy time to motivate myself to do it. Coming from a history of being sedentary, I can safely reassure you that this is possible for you too! I hate to admit it, but I was a couch potato when I was at home, and I am a homebody. I felt so heavy, physically and energetically, that I wouldn't do much of anything. I had no motivation whatsoever.

But then during this particular transformative year, after the break-up and doing all of the forgiveness work, belief work, intuitive eating, and intermittent fasting, my body started screaming for me to exercise.

I was walking my dog, Ceba, in the park one day. At that time, she was sixteen years old and still spunky. She would get these bursts of energy and just start running, and of course, like the good dog mom that I am, I would run with her.

But on this particular day, I felt and heard my body telling me in no uncertain terms: "You need to start jogging!" It was clear as day, and I made the decision at that moment. I would start jogging, something that I had always said I hated, and would never do. Jogging in particular was something I would judge others for doing when it was cold out, saying, "Those people are crazy."

It was fall at this time, and starting to get chilly, but I was determined because I could not ignore the desire my body had so clearly expressed. So I started jogging at the park. I didn't want people to see me jog because I felt uncomfortable, and like a fraud. I felt embarrassed because I knew I was going to be slow. But I was committed.

I started out by greeting the park when I entered. Hello, trees! Hello birdies! Hello, sky! Hello, lake! Hello, earth! Hello, air! Thank you all so much for being here and holding me. Remember, I was going through a break-up at this time, so I also needed to connect with the healing aspect of nature as well. Nature symbolized trusting the divine energy that was surrounding me.

As I would try to motivate myself to start jogging, I heard my mind say things like, "I don't want to jog," "There's no way I'm going to get around the lake," "I don't feel like doing this," "I'm tired," and numerous other sabotaging thoughts.

So I focused my mind and came up with other thoughts that felt better and truer. "You just have to run for short spurts," "You can always take a break when you get tired," "You're just starting, and it's going to take time to build this jogging muscle," "You got this!"

So I just started jogging, and trust me when I tell you, it was hard. I could only jog for a minute at a time before losing my breath, but I timed my walking break and started jogging again when the alarm went off.

Eventually, on my first day, I made it around the lake! I took too many breaks to count, but I did it. That was a huge accomplishment for me, and I celebrated!

I decided I wanted to jog three times a week. I set up my goals and did the work to get my butt to the park. Over time and with a lot of patience and the right mindset, I started to pick up my speed and could run longer durations without stopping. I was amazed by how fast my body was getting conditioned and I was so proud of myself for showing up. Eventually I was able to run around the entire park (3.35 miles) stopping only two or three times! I decided to get even more inspiration by signing up for a 5k race with my friend who is an experienced runner, and we started training together once a week.

She taught me more about body alignment and sprinting in order to condition my lungs and to improve my time. Thanks to her tips, I was able to run around the park without stopping, and the 'killer' hill didn't 'kill' me anymore! It was a powerful experience to give myself a chance at winning by trusting the process and knowing that it was going to take time, practice, and lots of self-compassion for me to reach my goal of running a ten-minute mile. I never hit that goal at the race – it was around 10:30 – but I started at a twelve-minute mile, and that was huge. Getting around the park without stopping was huge, and it still is.

Let yourself take in how good it feels to take care of yourself. The pride you feel when you make a choice that you may not have made in the past. If you don't feel motivated to exercise, get yourself turned-on first. Do a dance break, put on a cute workout outfit, pump yourself up with mirror work.

If you are still having a challenging time getting yourself to exercise, I suggest connecting with a buddy and doing fun things like Zumba classes, speed walking in the park, yoga, trampolining, or going out to dance or salsa class. This is all about meeting yourself where you are and finding the pleasure in it. You will create momentum as you go, as I did with jogging, so start somewhere that feels doable for you with the intention of increasing your intensity and quantity.

EXERCISE MIRROR WORK RITUAL

If you have access to a mirror, put it in front of your workout station at home or look at yourself in the mirror at the gym. Look at yourself as if you are your own trainer, cheering and coaching yourself through the workout the entire time. Look in your eyes and tell yourself how amazing you are and how you're killing it. Visualize yourself as the athlete you are or whatever you desire to be and believe it.

See yourself as your future self now. See yourself as whatever you desire to be now. If your desire is to feel alive and energized, you can visualize yourself with the glow oozing out of you already. See it in your minds eye. If you desire to run a 5k, visualize yourself running that race. If you desire to feel sexy walking down the street, visualize that. Look straight into your eyes and soul and see yourself as that person. Drop right into that vision. Let your vision fuel your exercise and let the intensity of the exercise fuel your vision.

This future self is who you are now. She's inside of you already; she just hasn't come out on the physical level yet. She's in the energetic desire realm. But that doesn't make her less real.

When you are finished exercising, take a moment to thank yourself, your loved ones on the other side, and your higher power for holding space for this alchemical journey.

FEAR BURNING RITUAL

As you begin to sweat as you intensify your exercise, imagine the fear, shame, and any emotion that has been living in your body armor being burned out as you exercise. This is an alchemical process that requires you to use your focus, your imagination, and your cultivated ability to feel.

Feel and visualize the emotions being released out of your fat, your cells, your being, as you increase your heart rate and sweat. You are moving the stuck energies that have been residing inside of your system, releasing the emotional weight that has been holding you down. Let the intensity of the exercise fuel your focus and let your focus fuel your intensity.

When you are finished exercising, take a moment to thank yourself, your loved ones on the other side, and your higher power for holding space for this alchemical journey.

Not living in your potential is the thing that makes you feel depleted, stuck, and tired. That includes our physical potential. Your energy (yang) needs to be used by movement. Your blood (yin) needs to be nourished by food. Your entire self needs quality sleep to integrate. When you don't honor this foundational truth, you don't give yourself the opportunity to live your best life. It blocks your channels to the source energy, which includes creativity, love, financial abundance, and intimacy in relationships. It takes a certain level of courage to listen, trust, and act accordingly. The question is if you're willing to do things differently.

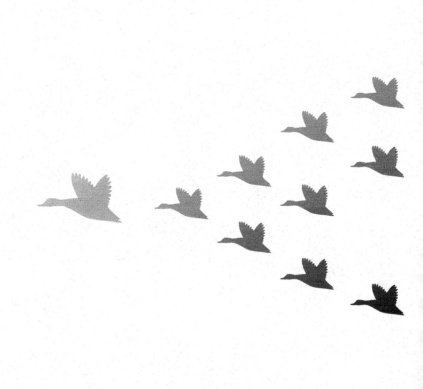

CHAPTER 11

ADULTING 101

"Awareness without action is like sitting in a poopy diaper."
— Unknown

always prided myself on being a free bird and doing what I wanted, when I wanted. That's partly why I've worked for myself for almost twenty years. I needed freedom and to be fluid. But here's the thing: I found out that I actually crave fluidity *and* structure. I noticed that when I have structure, I not only follow through more, but I experience more flow. The structure provides the freedom to flow. You will find that as you create a clear container for yourself, you will feel more at ease and more inspired to take action.

Structure and discipline are considered dirty words in some healing communities. Everyone is so focused on being connected to the yin that they tend to disregard the yang. As you are well aware of by this point, I honor and respect both energies, and I am clear that they both need to exist in our process as equals, and in tandem with each other. The internal yin work is just as important as the external yang work. The yin flow is just as important as the yang structure.

GOAL SETTING

Goal setting is a powerful tool. It sets you up for success by aligning you to your desire, while having a plan so you can take massive action in whatever ways make the most sense for you. Goal setting empowers you to go for it! It supports you in staying accountable to yourself. Goals are like that nagging best friend that won't let you off the hook when you tell them your biggest dream.

Goal Setting was the tool I needed to get myself into shape – literally and figuratively. To be able to see on paper what it was that I envisioned for myself and the steps I needed to get there. It was a potent reality check, and one that I needed, welcomed, but also rolled my eyes at in the moments I wanted to give up. But thank goddess for this tool because I honestly don't know if I would've been able to follow through without putting my goals on paper and returning back to work with them every single day.

When I began my weight releasing journey, I got clear on what it was that I desired for myself, my big 'why?', and the actions that needed to be taken to get there. Here's the except from my first goal setting process:

Big goal: Shed my body armor, specifically 20 pounds in 13 weeks.

My why: Because I want to experience the feeling of confidence from having completed something that historically has been challenging for me.

Progress goals:

1. Release 1.5 pounds per week
2. Jog 12 minutes per mile
3. Go to bed by midnight

Actions:

For Progress Goal #1
- Intermittent fasting
- Eat out once a week max
- Cut out ice cream

For Progress Goal #2
- Jog 3x/ week around the park
- Jogging sprints 1x/ week
- Trampoline 2x/ week

For Progress Goal #3
- Start night-time ritual after walking Ceba
- Stop screens at 10 p.m.
- Listen to Yoga Nidra meditation every night in bed

As I continued this process, and got to know myself better, I made various adjustments to the actions. It was a true time of discovery. I learned that I could depend on myself in this new physical form; that my word to myself was full of integrity; and when I was unable to rise to the occasion, I practiced being kind to myself. And choose to start fresh again.

GOAL SETTING RITUAL

- *Begin by writing out all of the desires you have for your body for at least 10 minutes. Don't overthink it. Just let yourself do a brain dump. Write everything that you desire no matter how confronting or silly it might feel. Let yourself feel the release of moving all of that energy from your brain to the paper.*
- *Now review all of the desires you listed and pick the top three desires.*
- *From those three, pick the number one top priority.*
- *Write out what measurable goal can happen in the next 13 weeks. Make it as specific as possible. For example: releasing 1.5 pounds a week or jogging a twelve-minute mile.*
- *Then write down all of the actions you need to take to reach that goal. Brain dump here again.*
- *Pick the top three actions that feel the most impactful and realistic for you in this moment.*
- *Schedule those actions in your calendar and incorporate them into your life.*
- *Continue to check in with your goals and actions every day to keep you inspired and motivated.*

Now if you're a geek like me and love checking off boxes and like having a tool to keep you organized and accountable, you have to check out the Self Journal tool! www.bestself.co

Congratulations! You are now on your way to building new healthy habits.

CREATING HABITS

You've lived a certain way for most or all of your life, and now you're trying to do this completely differently. It can feel overwhelming if you see it that way or you can see it as creating shifts one day at a time. Something to keep in mind is that resistance creates self-sabotage. It's important to be aware of the common ways people are likely to halt their progress:

- Future-tripping about failing.
- Overdoing it by implementing too many new habits at once.
- Thinking that something else needs to be finished before beginning.
- Thinking that a resource is needed before beginning. For example: a gym membership, money, etc.
- Thinking that their body is broken and unable to exercise.

You'll know when you're sabotaging because you'll feel stuck and yucky. Being able to be radically honest with yourself, and call yourself out when you get glimmers of sabotage, will change the game because it actually feels good to have integrity with yourself.

I also find that it is necessary to redefine what self-care actually is. True self-care is not over indulgence. My client described it best: if a child were acting out, would you give them a cupcake? I'm thinking probably not! The same is true with you. Do you tell yourself that laying around all day in the house is being gentle with yourself when what you are really doing is avoiding and over- indulging? This is not to say that laying around the house is bad and should never happen. I'm pointing to a specific moment when you're in resistance, and instead of doing your best you choose to not do anything. I find that many women who are trying to release weight tend to conflate indulgence with being gentle. Indulgence is not being in tune with where you are in the moment, as it dishonors your needs and desires. Authentic gentleness asks that you be in tune with your needs and desires, while at the same time not letting yourself off the hook by letting resistance win.

When creating new habits, I recommend pairing each new habit with an existing habit. Here's some examples:

- You already make tea every morning but now you put your supplements next to the tea to trigger your memory.
- You already put lotion on your body after taking a shower but now you pair it with mirror work and self-pleasure rituals in the morning.
- You already brush your teeth at night but now you pair it with shutting down your screens right after you brush your teeth.

HABIT PAIRING RITUAL

- *Take out a pen and paper and draw a vertical line down the middle of the paper.*
- *On the left side, make a list of the healthy habits you currently have ingrained in your day to day living.*

- *On the right side, make a list of the habits you desire to integrate in your life.*
- *Scan both lists and see if there are any habits that can be paired together that makes sense as seen in examples above.*
- *There is no need to do this for all of the habits listed. It's just a starting point of building new habits and a positive mindset around habits in general.*

It's important to take it one step at a time and at your own pace. Don't try to make all the changes at once. Pick the thing that feels most accessible to you and stick with it. The more you stick with it, the more your confidence grows. And then you'll feel like you can do the next thing. You are creating your mindset every time you follow through with something that you didn't know you could do. Creating new habits is a mind game and about building momentum. So be strategic and smart about it. This is the time to use your intelligence!

The whole process of changing your lifestyle is the perfect research study to get to know yourself. So while you are practicing with your food, exercise, and sleep and other self-care routines, you are learning about yourself. This is not about only getting to the goal, but also about diagnosing and discovering along the way. You will learn about what works for you and what doesn't. And then you will adjust based on what you've learned. It's all research! That's life.

If you're feeling stuck and unmotivated, the best thing to do is shake it up a bit. Do something different than what you're currently doing. Move your body. Not necessarily exercise but move your body to get your breathing up as a way to change your state of mind. Jump up and down. Take deep intense breaths. Take a walk outside. Take a shower. Just do something different.

Also, those moments are a good time to reset your intentions. Get really honest with yourself and ask yourself what your intention is for the next hour or so. This will keep you from spinning out into the future. One step at a time. Procrastination and feeling stuck happen when you're living in the future or ruminating on the past. So if you just focus on the moment and what you want to do in the immediate future, you will find that you are naturally building momentum.

Momentum is where it's at and that's why it's crucial for me to create a morning and night time ritual. Every time we go to sleep, our momentum stops. So in the morning, it's time to get the momentum going again. If I don't have a ritual to help me get my mind and body flowing, it will make the rest of the day more challenging and with more resistance. When I create my morning ritual, I make sure to pick a couple of things that will help me to create the right state of mind. A nighttime ritual is just as important because coming down pleasurably from the day means that your sleep will be more restorative, which means you are setting yourself up to have more energy and clarity for the following day.

CREATING A MORNING AND NIGHTTIME RITUAL

Here's a list practices for the morning and evening. Pick two for the morning and two for the night.

Morning practices:

- *Meditation*
- *Write in your journal*
- *Stretch or yoga*
- *Take a walk outside and connect with nature*
- *Dance break*
- *Mirror work*
- *Listening or reading something inspirational*

Nighttime practices:

- *Shut down screens two hours before sleep*
- *Write in your journal*
- *Stretch or yoga*
- *Take an Epsom salt bath with lavender essential oil*
- *Read a book*
- *Self-pleasure*
- *Listen to a guided sleep meditation*

DIGESTING YOUR BODY CHANGES

Digesting the changes that are happening to your body is as important as the actions taken to release the weight. Have you met people that released a bunch of weight but never felt comfortable in their new skin, so they unconsciously gained it all back? Or perhaps that was you at some point. Taking the weight back happens when the internal and external aspects of you are not in resonance. What I mean by this is that the inside has not caught up with the outside and a state of tangible, ongoing embodiment has not yet been reached. This is why I stress the importance of doing the internal work while we build a sustainable connection with our bodies along the way.

So do your mirror work and look at yourself with amazement about the shifts you have made, big and small. Look at all of you and see yourself with your love filters. See how beautiful you really are.

I personally love before and after photos, and I highly recommend them as a way to digest your body's transformation. Take a photo of your whole body from the front, back, and side angle and continue to take photos once a month. Then create side-by side-photos before and after photos with a photo editor for the front, side, and back angles. Then check yourself out and see all the small or big changes you've made in that time frame compared to the last photo. This is not an exercise to scrutinize yourself. This is an exercise to celebrate your wins!

Start to release your clothes that don't fit. As you release the weight, buy new clothes that express who you are at this point in your life. This will not only support you in digesting your new body, but you'll also feel this latent desire to own your sensual and sexual self and radiate your light. When a woman is able to own and embody their unique sensual nature, magic happens! When a woman owns her sensuality, she owns her power and light.

COMMUNITY

Practicing in a community is always beneficial. Not only will it add to your accountability, but it will also provide support when you are not feeling so hot. To be witnessed on your journey in a safe space is a transformative experience, especially when it comes to something so personal and protected as the fear fat suit. Allow yourself to be vulnerable and share what's happening for you: share your emotions, your well-earned wins, and definitely your failures, disappointments, and bumps on the road. Also, through witnessing other people on their journeys you can be reminded that you are not alone, that your problems are not unique. Finally, you'll be inspired to keep going. It's a win-win!

THE OTHER SIDE

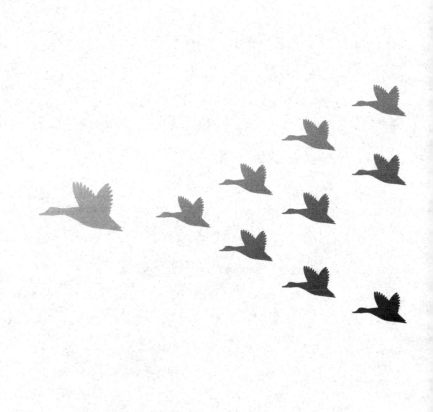

CHAPTER 12

FLOW

"Life is a series of natural and spontaneous changes. Don't resist them - that only creates sorrow. Let reality be reality. Let things flow naturally forward in whatever way they like."
— Lao Tzu

You have now walked through the yin and yang portals. You have completed many rituals, meditations, and exercises. I'm proud of you and I hope you feel proud too! I'm imagining that you're discovering all kinds of things about yourself. You're recovering old memories, getting reacquainted with your inner child and all the gifts and dreams you once had. You're feeling a lot more connected to your body, releasing stories that no longer serve you and having breakthrough after breakthrough. This has been a process of you practicing trusting yourself to hold space for you. And now you are expanding your capacity to be even more present and receptive by bringing flow into your everyday life.

Yay! Now what?

Now you stir it all in a pot and mix it up! Mix all the practices up and allow yourself to experiment by combining the emotional, mental, and physical rituals together along with everything else you've learned. You are exploring and experimenting in both new and wondrous ways that are unique to *your* personal flow. Experiment with listening to your internal guiding system and have fun with it. Continue to play with all of the elements you have been introduced to. Make it a game.

Have you ever watched a surfer catching waves? That's flow. They are having the time of their life while being so attuned to nature and what each moment is being asked of them. Being able to ride the energetic yin and yang waves will allow you to be in harmony with the same flow states as that surfer. When you tap into this mysterious, invisible, energetic realm, you open yourself up to living at one with source energy.

In Chinese medicine, if there's no flow it means that stagnant energy and/or disease are present. In order to unblock the stuck energy and create movement in our lives, we need to connect with this unseen world and learn how to be *with* it. And that's exactly what you've been cultivating while doing the practices in this book. You are increasing your ability to feel, be present, and connect to your body, mind, and spirit. These new found skills will support you in harnessing the energetic connections that will unite you with your flow.

To be in flow requires:

- Presence: Being present to feel, hear, or see the intuitive whispers and 'knowings' that arise in you.

- Trust: *Trust those 'knowings'.*
- Action: *Follow through with what those whispers are telling you.*

Flow is one hundred percent about being present with the reality of this moment. When you release your attachments to your expectations and your ways of trying to control life, flow automatically happens. You don't have to work to be in flow. The energy is moving with or without you, but if you choose to flow, you will find that your quality of life will increase exponentially. When you are gripping onto fear and trying to manipulate situations to be the way you want them to be, you have taken yourself out of flow. You know when you are flowing when life feels fluid, clear, and like it's happening organically, with ease, and you're exactly where you are supposed to be. This happens not only with "positive" situations, but is also true with painful ones. You can grieve and still be in flow. As a matter of fact, if you practice feeling your emotions, you will eventually be able to feel how good it feels to move through your pain while in flow.

BENEFITS OF FLOW

Experiencing greater intuition is the ultimate confirmation of your alignment in all the realms. You feel a sense of freedom because you are moving through life with a deep knowing that you are being guided, moment to moment, that living from a place of trusting your internal guiding system actually feels more secure than trying your old ways of grasping for security by attempting to control the outcome.

Can you imagine how good it would feel to do this with your body care? Trusting that you will know when to eat, what to eat, and when to stop eating; trusting that you will listen to your body's wisdom to get up and exercise or rest in the ways your body is craving; trusting that you can just check in and know where you are at this moment; trusting that you can get back into flow when you fall out of it.

When you trust the flow, you are connected to your truth. You trust what you're feeling so when you feel a truth arise in you, you trust that too. And being in tune with flow, you are able to speak that truth. There's such a cultivated connection with source energy that your clarity is grounded in you. There is no more questioning why you are here and what your purpose is because you know who you are. There's a sense of uprightness that takes over your body and energy, a satisfaction within yourself and living from what you know to be true.

When you trust the flow, you also trust yourself and the process. Women who have been hiding behind their weight and have tried to release it by only attempting to change their diet and exercise have lost their trust in the process and in themselves. When in flow, you know that you are doing your best and that your word holds power and integrity. You also are so much more loving to yourself and know that when you say you are going to do something that feels in alignment with what you desire, you do it and you surrender to the steps it takes to get there because you know that you can do whatever it is you put your mind to.

When you trust the organic flow of life, you naturally open up your receptivity. Most people move through life in defense mode, with one or more forms of shields. When you allow yourself to surrender to what is arising in you in every moment, you shed the protective barriers that prevent you from receiving love, your desires, attention, financial abundance, connection to self, and anything else. There's a feeling of openness and relaxation because you know that you are worthy of receiving all of the abundance you desire. There's a graciousness and ease that washes over you because there's no more fighting to get what you want.

Looking back on my life, I recall having so much abundance, whether it was loving support from friends, financial success, or supportive parents. But I was never satisfied because I wasn't allowing myself to receive any of the goodness coming my way. I always felt it was never enough, but that was just a reflection of what I thought about myself. I created many layers of "stay away" without even knowing it. But once I started to do the work of loving myself, through the entry points, I was able to receive all of the love around me and in me.

When people talk about receiving, usually they are referring to objects associated with cultural definitions of wealth and success: cars, jobs, relationships, and money, but as you start to build your receiving muscles, you will find that the most precious gift is a new ability to receive love, not only from other people but most importantly from yourself and the Universe, receiving it because there's a new and expanded level of trust in you that you no longer need to defend.

Being connected to your flow is another way of saying that you are at one with source energy. It means that you have no doubt about your connection to the divine and all of the abundance it provides. It means that you are surrendered to the miraculous unfolding of your life and know that the Universe has your back. You no longer question what it means to feel connected to the energy that connects all living and non-living beings.

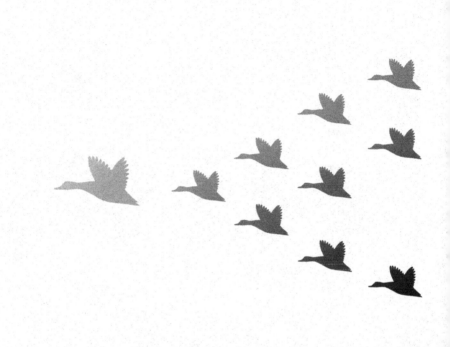

CHAPTER 13

YOU ARE YOUR OWN ARTWORK

"Our deepest fear is not that we are inadequate. Our deepest fear is that we are powerful beyond measure. It is our Light, not our Darkness, that most frightens us."
— Marianne Williamson

I believe our purpose in life is to radiate our own unique light in the world. This process of releasing weight is not only about shedding fat – it's about shedding the protective barriers that hide our light because at one point or another in your life, you took on a belief that it's not safe to be a radiant glowing goddess.

When I fell in love with my body and released my fear fat suit, I had this moment while walking to the train station. I was feeling like a million bucks, and I heard a whisper in my mind that said, "You are your own artwork." This is what I mean by radiance is purpose. You can work in any field, even if it doesn't feel like your true calling, but still feel connected to who you truly are. You are already living your purpose when you are glowing from the inside out.

Here's the secret: when you are radiating like this, you will be divinely guided to the work that is your calling.

It's the owning and honoring of who you are that allows you to be a shining star, shining so bright that you inspire everyone who is in your presence. Whether you say something or not doesn't matter. They will feel you oozing with light and that light is love and can cause the most powerful ripple effects. So even if you're in a "dead-end job," you will be creating ripples of love. This is how I believe we can change the world, one person at a time.

When you own this truth, you can embody it. Let that truth sink into how you move, walk, talk, exercise, eat, work, make love. You can make a choice to let what has shifted on the inside (self-love) come out to express itself on the outside.

What I noticed a couple of months into my journey was that I started to walk differently, partly because my body was changing and becoming more physically aligned and partly because I was feeling so good on the inside. One day, I caught myself walking down the street, and I felt like I was gliding. I was upright, and my head was held high. I had a pep in my step, and my hips were swaying from side to side.

I used to be the type of person who didn't want attention. I mean I did, but I didn't. I didn't feel safe, so I did my typical invisibility cloak thing by not making eye contact and by dressing myself down. I had a challenging time receiving attention, and when I got attention, I would shut down internally by either pretending to be confident like I wasn't fazed by the attention or just going small. But when you radiate, you feel safe in your body, with yourself, and with others. You feel safe everywhere!

OWN YOUR GLOW RITUAL

I invite you to feel the yumminess of your body when you're walking down the street. Feel your body. Feel the alignment in your spirit. Feel the alignment of your spine. Open your chest and your heart. Connect with your muscles while moving. Feel your hips swing. Feel energy and electricity moving through your body. Make eye contact with strangers. Perhaps give them a little smile or a shimmery eye twinkle. Offer them the gift of seeing the beauty of love that lives within you. You are an embodied goddess. There's no need to hide it anymore.

CHAPTER 14

CONCLUSION

"The journey of a thousand miles begins with one step."
— Lao Tzu

I wrote this book because I have experienced the power of shedding my fear fat suit and how that has completely changed my life in every way, shape, and form. I now know how it feels to be truly alive and living a life on purpose after a lifetime of suffering. My intention in writing this book is to inspire you and others to choose the path of self-realization.

I wrote this book for the little girl in me that was scared and hiding, and for the little girl in you that wants to be seen and share her highest version of herself into the world. It's such a gift for me to be able to share this with you, as it has created deeper healing for myself. My hope is that this book will have a ripple effect and continue to create deeper healing for you and the world.

I believe we all have a light burning bright within us already, but we just need to shed the layers that are hiding it. These security blankets are creating a false sense of safety. When I felt the elation and love arise in me while releasing my physical and emotional weight, I saw the real me for the first time.

I was able to own exactly who I am with no more shame, invisibility cloaks, or body armor. I was able to let people see the deepest and most true parts of me that always wanted to be seen. I became more generous with my heart, with strangers, friends, and family because I no longer was in survival mode. I touched my biggest desire of being able to love another human unconditionally for the first time because I fell in love with myself.

I became a woman of true faith, and even in the course of losing one loved one after another, I was able to stay connected to my knowledge of what is true.

With all of this bursting out of me, I could not keep it to myself. It had to be shared for others to receive. It has been quite an adventure for me to translate my internal process into something as concrete as words, and now coming to the end of it, it feels quite surreal. We have covered so much territory, and I am so honored that you have made it all the way to the end.

As you transform yourself, you will transform your life, and a natural outcome of that is you will feel inspired to pay it forward. That can happen with a smile to a stranger or sharing your story. Whatever it is that calls to you, I urge you to listen and do it. This life moves fast if we are not present, and we have the ability to slow down to choose connection to self and to others. Shine your unique light which is the highest level of expression of you, And in return, receive all the abundance that is magnetized to you.

This is the beauty of this life-changing journey: When you are connected to source energy you will never be able to withhold your light anymore. Take this process into your life and wrap your arms around it, embrace it. Live in the rituals and keep coming back to the practice every day. If you need reminders or inspiration along the way, revisit chapters that are calling out to you, call a friend on the path, or contact me for support.

You have opened the door to this brave new world, and it's time to step through. Don't turn back. Keep walking toward that light that already lives within you and be generous in sharing the gifts you hold.

Our personal transformations are a reflection of society's transformation. The more we heal ourselves, the more humanity heals. Be a direct warrior of change by doing the work on yourself first and foremost. The world needs it.

"You must be the change you wish to see in the world."
— Mahatma Gandhi

ACKNOWLEDGMENTS

This book would not have happened if it weren't for the loss of my last relationship and the crossing over of my dog, Ceba, and my cat, Baby. This all happened in three months' time, to the day, and it was a painful yet magical journey of loss to creation. I got to see up close and personal how the Universe works when you alchemize your pain into unconditional love. I am grateful for the profound experience this has been and continues to be in me stepping into the next era of my life.

I am so grateful for my Ma, who modeled what a powerful and service-oriented leader is — a woman that takes risks, follows her intuition, and lives a life of exploration. Rest in peace and in power, Ma. And for my Ba, who has downloaded his wisdom in me starting in the laundromat. A man who has guided me with complete and utter unconditional love and never judged me even in my darkest moments, the most loving space holder I know. And my stepfather, Sifu, who was inspired me to be a Chinese medicine practitioner and energy worker. His compassion and ability to connect with energy medicine was such a gift for me to experience firsthand. Rest in peace and in power, Sifu. And all of my ancestors, furry family and human friends who I feel guiding me, from the other side, every day.

To all of my teachers along the way, whether a mentor in a course, a stranger on the street, or a person I had a challenging relationship with. I am grateful that our paths crossed at one point or another and for all the clarity I have received from our connection.

To Alicia Muñoz for your unique and magical ability to see me and others so deeply. You are a brilliant and gifted writer and I am so grateful that you shared that gift through your beautiful, eloquent words in my foreword.

To my beloved friends that have loved me so deeply and supported me through the years. You know who you are. Thank you for the gift of sisterhood. It means the world to me. I love you.

To Barrie Cole who edited this book with her gift of wordsmithing and feeling what I desired to express. You rock!

To the crew that helped me to create an amazing photo for this book. Nancy La Lanne of La Lanne Photography (photographer), Odu Adamu (stylist), Melinda Bouldin owner of Heritage Hair NYC (hair stylist), and Isabelle DeRose (makeup artist). Thank you for bringing your talents and joy!

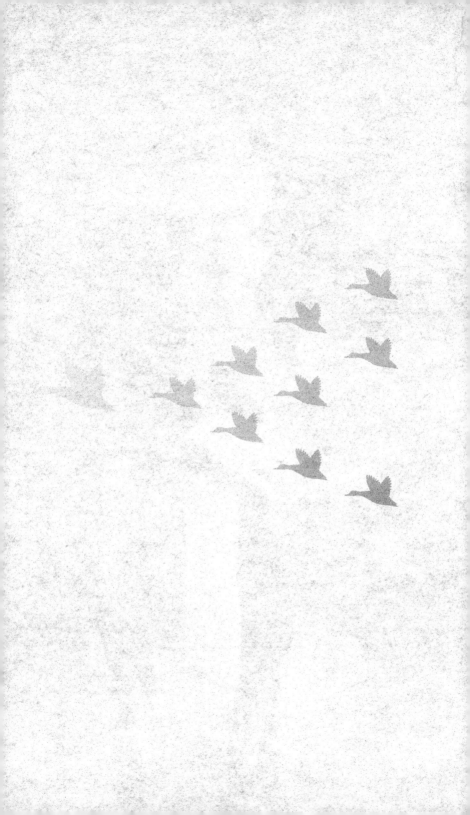

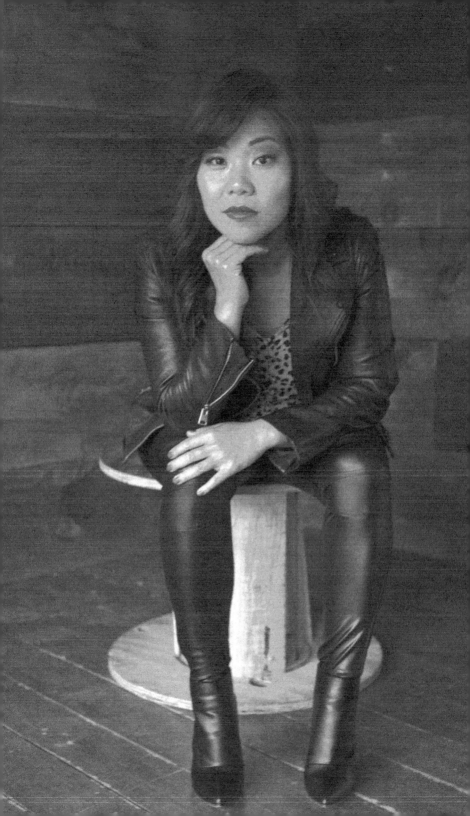

ABOUT THE AUTHOR

P O - H O N G Y U is an acupuncturist, coach, and energy practitioner. She brings a mixture of her personal healing experiences, her intuitive and empathic gifts, and her extensive professional experiences to support women who are ready to reclaim their bodies and their power.

She passionately believes that healing happens from the inside out and guides women to face and release their fears in order to be a beacon of light in the world. s

Po-Hong is a shadow and lightworker and uses her ability to focus her attention and feel her client's energy blockages as a way to help usher them into their next level of freedom.

She is radical in that she honors and gives thanks to her childhood traumas. She views them as gifts and portals into the deeper healing path that she traveled and, as a result, has expanded her capacity to hold others in their shadows. On the other end of the spectrum, her ability to connect with source energy has given her the gift of faith in the divine and the ability to hold the vision of what's possible for her clients.

Po-Hong received her MS in acupuncture at Tri-State College of Acupuncture in NYC and her BA in psychology from

Temple University in Philadelphia. She became a life coach through the OneTaste coaching program, which is based on the principles of energetic flow states.

She lives happily in Brooklyn, NY and travels through life with a childlike curiosity and a burning desire to make a difference in the world. She is continuously expanding her knowledge by taking a variety of courses and staying open to life's lessons.

You can find her at www.thelightactivator.com.

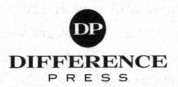

ABOUT DIFFERENCE PRESS

Difference Press is the exclusive publishing arm of The Author Incubator, an educational company for entrepreneurs – including life coaches, healers, consultants, and community leaders – looking for a comprehensive solution to get their books written, published, and promoted. Its founder, Dr. Angela Lauria, has been bringing to life the literary ventures of hundreds of authors–in–transformation since 1994.

A boutique–style self–publishing service for clients of The Author Incubator, Difference Press boasts a fair and easy–to–understand profit structure, low–priced author copies, and author–friendly contract terms. Most importantly, all of our #incubatedauthors maintain ownership of their copyright at all times.

LET'S START A MOVEMENT WITH YOUR MESSAGE

In a market where hundreds of thousands of books are published every year and are never heard from again, The Author Incubator is different. Not only do all Difference Press books reach Amazon bestseller status, but all of our authors are actively changing lives and making a difference.

Since launching in 2013, we've served over 500 authors who came to us with an idea for a book and were able to write it and get it self–published in less than 6 months. In addition, more than 100 of those books were picked up by traditional publishers and are now available in book stores. We do this by selecting the highest quality and highest potential applicants for our future programs.

Our program doesn't only teach you how to write a book – our team of coaches, developmental editors, copy editors, art directors, and marketing experts incubate you from having a book idea to being a published, bestselling author, ensuring that the book you create can actually make a difference in the world. Then we give you the training you need to use your book to make the difference in the world, or to create a business out of serving your readers.

ARE YOU READY TO MAKE A DIFFERENCE?

You've seen other people make a difference with a book. Now it's your turn. If you are ready to stop watching and start taking massive action, go to <u>http://theauthorincubator.com/apply/</u>.

<u>"Yes, I'm ready!"</u>

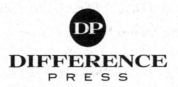

OTHER BOOKS BY
DIFFERENCE PRESS

So, You Want to Be a Superintendent?: Become the Leader You Were Meant to Be by Donna Marie Cozine Ed.D.

Outsmart Endometriosis: Relieve Your Symptoms and Get Your Career Back on Track by Jessica Drummond DNC, CNS, PT

Teach and Go Home: The Sophisticated Guide to Simplifying and Managing Your Workload and More by Danielle E. Felton

The Wealthy Entrepreneur: The Formula for Making Money and Gaining Financial Clarity in Your Business by Robert Gauvreau FCPA

TMJ Is Ruining My Life: Managing Jaw Pain so You Can Eat Normally by Chelsea Liebowitz PharmD, MSCR

My Child's Not Depressed Anymore: Treatment Strategies That Will Launch Your College Student to Academic and Personal Success by Melissa Lopez Larson M.D.

The 9 Pillars of the YONIVERSE: Attract Amazing Clients as a Female Tantric Practitioner by Palki Mawar

Evolved NLP: The Impact-Driven Coach's Guide to Amplified Revenue and Results by Laura Slinn, Kelley Oswin RSW, and Ernie Pavan

Death Is Not Goodbye: Connect with Your Loved Ones Again by Kim Weaver

The Happy, Healthy Revolution: The Working Parent's Guide to Achieve Wellness as a Family Unit by Theresa Wee M.D.

Reprogram Your Sleep: The Sleep Recipe that Works by Tara Youngblood